Monographs in Allergy (ISSN 0077–0760), **Vol. 28**
Series Editors: L.Å. Hanson, Göteborg; F. Shakib, Nottingham

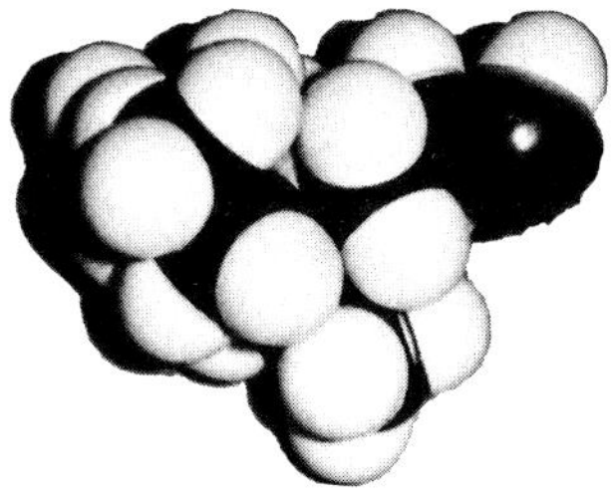

Editor: B.A. Baldo

Molecular Approaches to the Study of Allergens

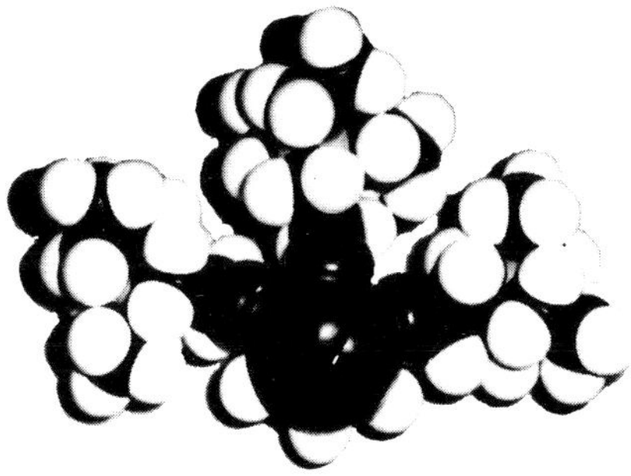

Unprecedented depth of coverage on the nature of allergenic determinants

There is a dearth of information available in the literature on the molecular aspects of allergens of all types from small molecules to large molecular weight proteins. This is the first book entirely devoted to the immunochemical and molecular biology of these allergy-causing agents and is also the first to provide a comprehensive overview of recombinant DNA methodology applied to allergens. Invited experts describe in detail the allergenic groupings identified on drugs implicated in allergic reactions, thoroughly discuss insect venom, rye-grass pollen, and Chironomid hemoglobin allergens, and highlight priorities in house dust mite research.

Enhanced by clear figures and tables, this unique single source contains original findings and powerful methodologies of great interest to allergists, clinical immunologists and researchers in molecular biology, immunology and protein chemistry.

Contents

Fields of Interest

Allergy, Immunology; Respiratory System; Asthma, Biochemistry, Molecular Biology, Pharmacology, Serology

Monographs in Allergy, Vol. 28
Molecular Approaches to the Study of Allergens
Editor: Baldo, B.A. (St. Leonards, N.S.W.)
VIII + 166 p., 38 fig., 33 tab., hard cover, 1990
SFr. 213.– / DM 255.– / £ 92.60 / US$ 170.50
US $ price for USA, £ price for UK only (subject to change)
ISBN 3–8055–5213–0

KARGER

Respiration

International Review of Thoracic Diseases

Founded 1944 as 'Schweizerische Zeitschrift für Tuberkulose und Pneumonologie' by E. Bachmann, M. Gilbert, F. Häberlin, W. Löffler, P. Steiner and E. Uehlinger, continued 1962–1967 as 'Medicina Thoracalis'

General Information

Publication data: 'Respiration' is published 6 times annually. Volume 58 with 6 issues appears in 1991.

Subscription rates: Subscriptions run for a full calendar year. Prices are given per volume, surface postage included.

Personal subscription: SFr. 359.80, US$ 288.40. (Must be in the name of, billed to, and paid by an individual. Order must be marked 'personal subscription'.)

Institutional subscription: SFr. 514.–, US$ 412.00. (Regular rate.)

Members of the European Society of Pneumology: SFr. 257.–, US$ 206.00.

Airmail postage: SFr. 35.–, US$ 25.00. (Extra per volume.)

Microform subscription: SFr. 257.–, US$ 206.00. (Available exclusively to subscribers of the paper edition.)

Single issues and back volumes: Information on availability and prices can be obtained through the Publisher.

Subscription orders: Orders can be placed at agencies, bookstores, directly with the Publisher S. Karger AG, P.O. Box, CH-4009 Basel (Switzerland) or with any of the following distributors:

Deutschland, Österreich, Ost-Europa: S. Karger GmbH, Postfach 1724, D-W-8034 Germering/München

France: Librairie Luginbühl, 36, bd de Latour-Maubourg, F-75007 Paris

Great Britain, Ireland: S. Karger Publishers, 1 Torberry Drive, Petersfield, Hampshire GU31 4HW

USA: S. Karger Publishers, Inc., 26 West Avon Road, P.O. Box 529, Farmington, CT 06085

India, Bangladesh, Sri Lanka: S. Karger India Subscription Agency, B-5/132 Safdarjung Enclave, New Delhi-110029

Japan: Katakura Libri, Inc., 36-9 Hongo 3-chome, Bunkyo-ku, Tokyo 113

Change of address: Both old and new address should be stated and sent to the subscription source.

Bibliographic indices: This journal is regularly listed in bibliographic services, including *Current Contents®*.

Book Reviews: Books are accepted for review by special agreement.

Advertising: Correspondence and rate requests should be addressed to the Publisher.

KARGER

Respiration
Printed in Switzerland

S. Karger AG,
Postfach, CH-4009 Basel (Schweiz)

Erscheint zweimonatlich;
pro Jahr 1 Band zu 6 Heften

Respiration

Submission: Original papers written in English, German or French will be considered but articles in English are preferred. They should be sent to:
S. Karger AG
Editorial Dept. 'Respiration'
P.O. Box
CH–4009 Basel (Switzerland)
Manuscripts should be submitted in triplicate (with three sets of illustrations of which one is an original), typewritten double-spaced on one side of the paper, with a wide margin.

Conditions: All manuscripts are subject to editorial review. Manuscripts are received with the explicit understanding that they are not under simultaneous consideration by any other publication. Submission of an article for publication implies the transfer of the copyright from the author to the publisher upon acceptance. Accepted papers become the permanent property of 'Respiration' and may not be reproduced by any means, in whole or in part, without the written consent of the publisher. It is the author's responsibility to obtain permission to reproduce illustrations, tables, etc. from other publications.

Arrangement:

Title page: The first page of each paper should indicate the title (main title underlined), the authors' names, and the institute where the work was conducted. A short title for use as running head and a translation of the complete title into English are also required.

Key words: For indexing purposes, a list of 3–10 key words in English is essential.

Abstract: Each paper needs an abstract of up to 10 lines in English and a summary of not more than 20 lines in the original language.

Small type: Paragraphs which can or must be set in smaller type (case histories, test methods, etc.) should be indicated with a 'p' (petit) in the margin on the left-hand side.

Footnotes: Avoid footnotes. When essential, they are numbered consecutively and typed at the foot of the appropriate page.

Tables and illustrations: Tables and illustrations (both numbered in Arabic numerals) should be prepared on separate sheets. Tables require a heading and figures a legend, also prepared on a separate sheet. For the reproduction of illustrations, only good drawings and original photographs can be accepted; negatives or photocopies cannot be used. When possible, group several illustrations on one block for reproduction (max. size 176 × 224 mm) or provide crop marks. On the back of each illustration, indicate its number, the author's name, and 'top'. Color illustrations are reproduced at the author's expense.

References: In the text identify references by Arabic numerals [in square brackets]. Material submitted for publication but not yet accepted should be noted as 'unpublished data' and not be included in the reference list. The list of references should include only those publications which are cited in the text. Do not alphabetize; number references in the order in which they are first mentioned in the text. The surnames of the authors followed by initials should be given. There should be no punctuation other than a comma to separate the authors. Cite all authors, 'et al' is not sufficient. Abbreviate journal names according to the Index Medicus system. (Also see International Committee of Medical Journal Editors: Uniform requirements for manuscripts submitted to biomedical journals. Br Med J 1988;296:401–405.)

Examples

(a) Papers published in periodicals: Kauffman HF, van der Heide S, Beaumont F, Blok H, de Vries K: Class-specific antibody determination against *Aspergillus fumigatus* by means of the enzyme-linked immunosorbent assay. III. Comparative study: IgG, IgA, IgM ELISA titers, precipitating antibodies and IgE binding after fractionation of the antigen. Int Arch Allergy Appl Immunol 1986;80:300–306.

(b) Monographs: Matthews DE, Farewell VT: Using and Understanding Medical Statistics. Basel, Karger, 1985.

(c) Edited books: Hardy WD Jr, Essex M: FeLV-induced feline acquired immune deficiency syndrome: A model for human AIDS; in Klein E (ed): Acquired Immunodeficiency Syndrome. Prog Allergy. Basel, Karger, 1986, vol 37, pp 353–376.

SI-Units: Since the United States of America and other countries outside Europe where 'Respiration' is read, have not accepted the SI-System, authors using SI-Units should add the conventional units in brackets, for example: pO_2 = 10 kPa (75 mm Hg).

Full address: The exact postal address complete with postal code of the senior author must be given. If correspondence is handled by someone else, indicate this accordingly.

Further details: Authors may consult our leaflet 'Rules for the Preparation of Manuscripts', available on request from the Publisher, S. Karger AG, P.O. Box, CH–4009 Basel (Switzerland).

Page charges: There is no page charge for papers of 4 or fewer printed pages (including tables, illustrations and references). Each additional complete or partial page is charged to the author at SFr. 225.– / US$ 150.00. The allotted size of a paper is equal to approx. 12 manuscript pages (including tables, illustrations and references).

Galley proofs: Unless indicated otherwise, galley proofs are sent to the first-named author and should be returned with the least possible delay. Alterations made in galley proofs, other than the correction of printer's errors, are charged to the author. No page proofs are supplied.

Reprints: Order forms and a price list are sent with the galley proofs. Orders submitted after the issue is printed are subject to considerably higher prices. Allow five weeks from date of publication for delivery of reprints.

KARGER

Chronic Bronchitis in the 90's

Chronic Bronchitis in the 90's

Satellite Workshop
June 1, 1989, Salsomaggiore (Parma), Italy

Guest Editors
J.A. Nadel, San Francisco, Calif.
D. Olivieri, Parma

7 figures, 14 tables, 1991

KARGER

Respiration

Vol. 58, Supplement 1, 1991

S. Karger · Medical and Scientific Publishers
Basel · München · Paris · London · New York · New Delhi · Bangkok · Singapore · Tokyo · Sydney

Drug Dosage

The authors and the publisher have exerted every effort to ensure that drug selection and dosage set forth in this text are in accord with current recommendations and practice at the time of publication. However, in view of ongoing research, changes in government regulations, and the constant flow of information relating to drug therapy and drug reactions, the reader is urged to check the package insert for each drug for any change in indications and dosage and for added warnings and precautions. This is particularly important when the recommended agent is a new and/or infrequently employed drug.

Printed in Switzerland on acid-free paper by Basler Zeitung, Basel
ISBN 3-8055-5452-4

Contents

Respiration 1991;58(suppl 1):1

Foreword

Chronic bronchitis represents one of the most common disease of the airways, whose importance from the clinical, epidemiological and social point of views is often underestimated.

It is not yet completely known why it evolves towards bronchial obstruction and/or towards the destruction of the lung parenchyma. For this reason it is not yet exactly defined whether treatment should essentially modify mucus hypersecretion, for instance reducing airway inflammation, or instead prevent repeated bronchopulmonary infections.

Several different points of view exist among different European countries and the US regarding a common terminology for different forms of chronic airway inflammation to establish common guidelines for therapy.

The meeting held at Salsomaggiore (Parma) on June 1, 1989 has gathered many experts from both sides of the Atlantic for an exchange of opinions about the most relevant problems to be expected in the next decade. Ideas have been confronted based on practical experience matured in diverse countries in the last years.

The proceedings of the meeting gathered in this issue testify to the commitment of the authors who synthesized most efficiently their personal contributions and at the same time considered the work of other groups in their own country.

The Editors

Respiration 1991;58(suppl 1):3–5

0025–7931/91/0587–0003 $ 2.75/0

Role of Enzymes from Inflammatory Cells on Airway Submucosal Gland Secretion[1]

J.A. Nadel

Cardiovascular Research Institute and Departments of Medicine and Physiology, University of California, San Francisco, Calif., USA

Key Words. Submucosal gland secretion · Serine protease · Neutrophil elastase and cathepsin G · Mast cell chymase

Abstract. We examined the roles of enzymes from mast cells and from neutrophils in stimulating airway submucosal gland secretion. To avoid effects on surface epithelial cells and goblet cells, we studied a line of cultured bovine tracheal gland serous cells. We discovered that mast cell chymase and neutrophil elastase are the most potent secretagogues of airway submucosal glands described. Mast cell chymase markedly stimulated serous cell secretion in a concentration-dependent fashion with a threshold of 10^{-10} *M*, whereas tryptase had no effect. The response to 10^{-8} *M* chymase (1,530 ± 80% over baseline; mean ± SEM) was approximately 10-fold higher than that evoked by other agonists such as histamine and isoproterenol. Both neutrophil proteases also stimulated secretion in a concentration-dependent fashion with a threshold of $>10^{-10}$ *M*. Elastase was more potent than cathepsin G, causing a maximal secretory response of 1,810 ± 60% over baseline at 10^{-8} *M*. Secretion by the 3 proteases was noncytotoxic and required catalytically active enzymes. These findings suggest a potential role for neutrophil and mast cell proteases in the pathogenesis of increased and abnormal submucosal gland secretions in diseases associated with inflammation of the airways.

Introduction

Submucosal glands are the major sources of airway secretions, and many mediators act as secretagogues. However, concentrations in excess of 10^{-8} *M* of agonists such as prostaglandins, histamine, and beta-adrenergic agonists are required to induce secretory responses [1–3], and the maximal responses to these mediators is not great. Diseases where the release of mast cell mediators is implicated (e.g. asthma) and diseases with inflammatory cell infiltration of airways (e.g. asthma, bronchitis, cystic fibrosis) are associated with excessive airway secretions. Therefore, we have investigated the roles of mast cell and neutrophil enzymes on gland cell secretion. The present studies indicate that mast cell chymase, neutrophil elastase, and neutrophil cathepsin G are the most potent stimuli to airway submucosal gland secretion thus far described. These results suggest a role for these 3 enzymes in the pathogenesis of increased secretions associated with inflammatory diseases, and they suggest a strategy for treating the abnormal secretions.

Methods

Because proteases can release glycoconjugates from epithelial cell surfaces [4] and from goblet cells [5], and because our goal was to study effects isolated to gland cells, we studied a line of bovine tracheal gland serous cells cultured as described elsewhere [1, 6]. Cells were studied between passages 10 and 25. Cells were seeded at a density of 2×10^4 cells/cm^2 on tissue culture plastic coated with human placental collagen (15 µg/cm^2) in medium containing Dubelcco's modified Eagles' H21 medium, 40% Ham's F12 medium, 20% fetal calf serum, and 50 µg/ml gentamicin. Flasks were maintained at 37 °C in 5% CO_2/95% air. We changed the medium every 3 days.

On day 9, confluent monolayers were incubated with medium

[1] Supported in part by a Cystic Fibrosis Foundation Research Development Program grant.

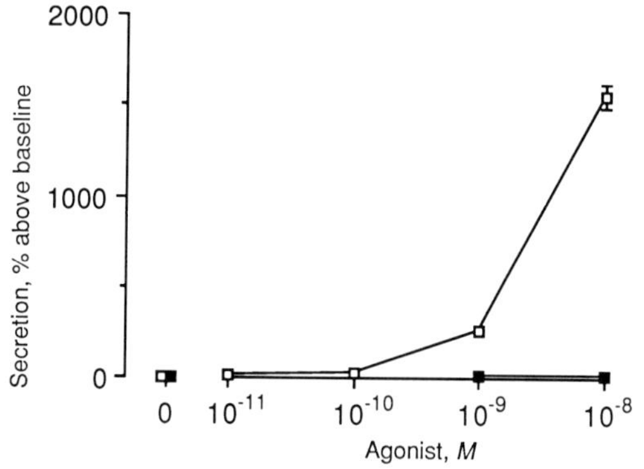

Fig. 1. Effect of chymase (□) and tryptase (■) on secretion of ^{35}S-labeled macromolecules from cultured tracheal gland serous cells. Secretion is greatly stimulated by chymase ($p < 0.0001$, $n = 5$), whereas tryptase has no significant effect. Values are mean ± SEM, n = 5 [6, reproduced with permission].

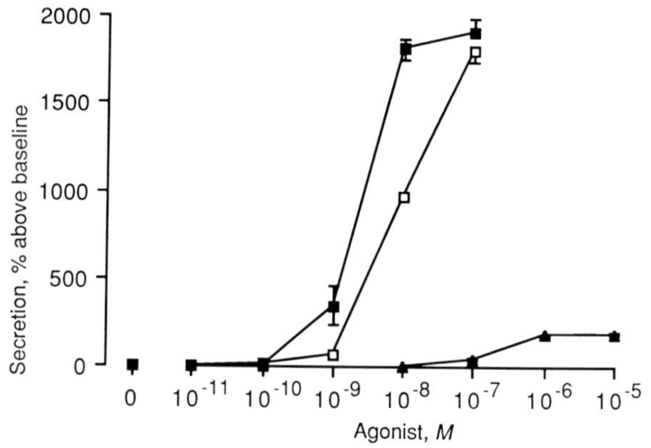

Fig. 2. Effects of human neutrophil cathepsin G (□) and elastase (■) and of histamine (▲) on secretion of ^{35}S-labeled macromolecules from cultured tracheal gland serous cells. Secretion is stimulated markedly by cathepsin G and elastase ($p < 0.0001$, $n = 5$), whereas histamine has a comparatively small effect ($p < 0.0001$, $n = 6$). Values are mean ± SEM [7, reproduced with permission].

containing $Na^{35}SO_4$, and the release of nondialyzable ^{35}S-labeled macromolecules was examined as described elsewhere [6, 7]. Mast cell chymase and tryptase were purified from dog mastocytoma cells [8, 9]. Human neutrophil elastase and cathepsin G isolated from human purulent sputum were purchased from Elastin Products (Pacific, Mo., USA).

Results

Mast Cell Enzyme

Purified tryptase had no significant effect on the release of ^{35}S-labeled macromolecules, but purified chymase caused a marked secretory response, with a threshold of 10^{-10} *M* (fig. 1) [6]. The response was concentration-dependent, and a maximal response was not achieved in the range of concentrations used (10^{-11}–10^{-8} *M*). The response to 10^{-8} *M* chymase (1,530 ± 80% over baseline; mean ± SEM) was approximately 10-fold higher than that evoked by other agonists such as histamine. The response to chymase was not due to a cytotoxic effect [6]. In the presence of soybean trypsin inhibitor (100 µg/ml) or chymostatin (10 µg/ml), the chymase-induced secretory response was inhibited or significantly reduced, indicating that the active catalytic site of the enzyme is required for its secretagogue activity.

In comparison to chymase, exogenous histamine also stimulated the secretion of ^{35}S-labeled macromolecules in a concentration-dependent fashion, but the threshold was higher ($\geq 10^{-8}$ *M*), and a plateau was achieved with a response of approximately 180% above baseline.

Neutrophil Enzymes

Human neutrophil cathepsin G and neutrophil elastase both stimulated secretion of ^{35}S-labeled macromolecules, with a threshold concentration of $\geq 10^{-10}$ *M* for both enzymes [7]. Secretion in response to both enzymes was concentration-dependent, but only the response to elastase reached a plateau with the concentrations used (10^{-11}–10^{-7} *M*). Elastase was more potent than cathepsin G, causing a maximal secretory response of 1,810 ± 60% above baseline (mean ± SEM) at 10^{-8} *M* (fig. 2). The protease-induced secretion was noncytotoxic and required catalytically active enzymes.

Discussion

These studies show that mast cell and neutrophil enzymes are the most potent secretagogues of airway submucosal gland secretion ever described. Our present information suggests that they cause secretion via a novel pathway and do not require receptor activation. In our studies, we chose cultured submucosal gland serous cells, so we could be sure that the secretion was derived from gland cells and not from surface epithelial cells or goblet cells.

Mast cell enzymes are major constituents of mast cell granules and amount to more than 20% of all protein in the cell. It is of interest that chymase, but not tryptase, is a potent secretagogue. This is significant because not all mast cells contain chymase. The presence of chymase-containing mast cells corresponds to the anatomic location of airway glands (i.e. they are concentrated in the submucosa of major airways [10]). Furthermore, in cystic fibrosis, a disease characterized by airway submucosal gland hypertrophy, chymase-containing mast cells in bronchoalveolar lavage are increased dramatically compared to normal subjects [11]. These findings suggest that chymase expression in mast cells may be influenced by the presence and activity of glands. The presence of chymase-containing mast cells in close association with airway submucosal glands and the extraordinary potency of chymase as a secretagogue suggest that mast cell chymase may play a significant role in the hypersecretion that is present in diseases such as asthma and cystic fibrosis. Furthermore, these facts suggest that an antagonist to chymase could make a significant contribution to the alleviation of the symptoms caused by hypersecretion in these diseases.

We have also studied the submucosal gland secretory responses to the enzymes released from a second inflammatory cell, the neutrophil. This cell produces the proteases elastase and cathepsin G. Similar to mast cell chymase, these 2 enzymes are potent secretagogues in submucosal gland serous cells, with maximal response approximately 10-fold larger than histamine and with low thresholds for responses, making them potentially powerful mechanisms for hypersecretion in inflammatory diseases. Because neutrophil elastase is a more potent secretagogue than cathepsin G, drugs that act as antagonists to elastase may be particularly useful in the therapy of inflammatory diseases of airways associated with hypersecretion.

In conclusion, enzymes that exist in granules of mast cells and of neutrophils are the most potent secretagogues of airway submucosal glands thus far described. Because these inflammatory cells are implicated in airway diseases associated with hypersecretion (e.g. cystic fibrosis, asthma, chronic bronchitis), antagonists to these enzymes could play important therapeutic roles in the treatment of hypersecretion in these diseases.

References

1 Finkbeiner WE, Nadel JA, Basbaum CB: Establishment and characterization of a cell line derived from bovine tracheal glands. In Vitro Cell Dev Biol 1986;22:561-567.
2 Sommerhoff CP, Finkbeiner WE, Nadel JA, Basbaum CB: Mediators of anaphylaxis stimulate ^{35}S-labeled macromolecule secretion from cultured bovine tracheal gland serous cells. Bull Eur Physiopathol Respir 1987;23:363s.
3 Sommerhoff CP, Finkbeiner WE, Nadel JA, Basbaum CB: Prostaglandin D_2 and prostaglandin E_2 stimulate ^{35}S-labeled macromolecule secretion from cultured bovine tracheal gland serous cells. Am Rev Respir Dis 1987;135:A363.
4 Varsano S, Basbaum CB, Forsberg LS, Borson DB, Caughey G, Nadel JA: Dog tracheal epithelial cells in culture synthesize sulfated macromolecular glycoconjugates and release them from the cell surface upon exposure to extracellular proteinases. Exp Lung Res 1987;13:157-183.
5 Kim KC, Wasano K, Niles RM, Schuster JE, Stone PJ, Brody JS: Human neutrophil elastase releases cell surface mucins from primary cultures of hamster tracheal epithelial cells. Proc Natl Acad Sci USA 1987;84:9304-9308.
6 Sommerhoff CP, Caughey CH, Finkbeiner WE, Lazarus SC, Basbaum CB, Nadel JA: Mast cell chymase: A potent secretagogue for airway gland serous cells. J Immunol 1989;142: 2450-2456.
7 Sommerhoff CP, Nadel JA, Basbaum CB, Caughey GH: Neutrophil elastase and cathepsin G stimulate secretion from cultured bovine airway gland serous cells. J Clin Invest 1990;85: 682-689.
8 Caughey GH, Viro NF, Lazarus SC, Nadel JA: Purification and characterization of dog mastocytoma chymase. Identification of an octapeptide conserved in chymotryptic leukocyte proteases. Biochim Biophys Acta 1988;952:142-149.
9 Caughey GH, Viro NF, Ramachandran J, Lazarus SC, Borson DB, Nadel JA: Dog mastocytoma tryptase: Affinity purification, characterization and amino-terminal sequence. Arch Biochem Biophys 1987;258:555-563.
10 Irani AA, Schechter NM, Craig SS, DeBlois G, Schwartz LB: Two types of human mast cells that have distinct neutral protease compositions. Proc Natl Acad Sci USA 1986;83:4464-4468.
11 Schwartz LB, Irani AA, Mroueh S, Spock A: Reversed ratio of T/TC types of human mast cells in cystic fibrosis. Clin Res 1987;35:255A.

Jay A. Nadel, MD
Cardiovascular Research Institute
Box 0130
University of California
San Francisco, CA 94143-0130 (USA)

Respiration 1991;58(suppl 1):6–9

0025–7931/91/0587–0006 $ 2.75/0

Chronic Bronchitis: Definition (Or Redefinition?)

P. Vermeire

Department of Respiratory Medicine, University of Antwerp, Belgium

Key Words. Chronic bronchitis, definition of · Chronic obstructive lung disease · Mucus secretion

Abstract. Although a quite precise clinical definition was given to the term 'chronic bronchitis' in the early sixties, the terminology related to nonasthmatic, nonemphysematous obstructive airway disease remains a continuous source of confusion, as indicated by a recent international survey. Although histological studies point to the presence of widespread bronchial inflammation in this condition, preference should be given to simple and descriptive terminology in which the presence of airflow limitation is clearly and predominantly indicated, since it mostly affects prognosis. There would be no need to redefine 'chronic bronchitis', but simply replacing it by 'chronic mucus hypersecretion', to which it actually refers, would be the preferred solution.

Purpose

The purpose of the present contribution to this Symposium is to briefly review definitions related to 'chronic bronchitis', the confusion generated by its terminology and to express some views as to what terminology should be carried into the nineties.

Definitions

Chronic bronchitis has been rather precisely defined by several authoritative scientific bodies [1–3] as the 'condition of subjects with chronic or recurrent hypersecretion of mucus into the bronchial tree', in which 'chronic or recurrent' was defined as 'occurring on most days for at least 3 months in the year during at least 2 years'. Obviously other bronchopulmonary disorders, such as bronchiectasis or tuberculosis, or cardiac disorders as sole cause for the symptoms needed to be excluded.

These defining criteria are entirely clinical and, unfortunately, do not indicate the presence of the frequently accompanying airway obstruction and consequent dyspnea on exertion. Because of the frequent association with chronic airway obstruction, it was also proposed in 1965 [3] to add qualifying labels, such as 'simple' (or nonobstructive) or 'obstructive' for a better definition of patients within the broad scope of chronic bronchitis; in some countries 'asthmatic' is also added to these qualifying labels when the obstructive component is markedly reversible and patients are suffering attacks of dyspnea and wheezing.

In practice, however, the term 'chronic bronchitis' is often used as a synonym for chronic airway obstruction. This confusion is based on the belief that there is a causal association between mucus hypersecretion and airway obstruction. However, morphological [4] and epidemiological [5] studies have demonstrated that mucus hypersecretion in central airways is not a cause of chronic airways obstruction; moreover, the latter may be severe without hypersecretion in central airways. It was therefore recommended [6] to abandon the term 'chronic bronchitis' – also because it wrongly suggests the presence of chronic infection – and to replace it by 'bronchial catarrh'.

With asthma and emphysema, chronic bronchitis was grouped by the 1959 Ciba Symposium [1] under 'chronic nonspecific lung diseases' (CNSLD), which could function as an 'umbrella' term for a number of diseases characterized by symptoms of breathlessness, cough and/or sputum production, not caused by localized or specific respiratory disease, nor by a disease of another organ system. This term was only adopted in Dutch-speaking countries under the term CARA (chronic aspecific respiratory affections) [7], where it also gives rise to misuse ('severe CARA patient') and misunderstandings if not adequately qualified.

The need for a better reference to the presence of chronic airway obstruction as a part of the disease process led to the use of additional umbrella terms like GOLD (generalized obstructive lung disease, i.e. CNSLD, excluding nonobstructive chronic bronchitis) or COPD (i.e. GOLD, excluding asthma), but the former term has never been adopted and the latter is unevenly used between countries. In France a similar term, BPCO (bronchopneumopathies chroniques obstructives), is widely used.

Confusion about Terminology

The confusion generated by terminology, in particular by the term 'chronic bronchitis', was well illustrated by two recent studies. In 1986, Dodge et al. [8] showed considerable bias in the diagnostic labeling by community physicians of 351 patients with quite similar clinical features of obstructive lung disease. Younger patients were more likely to be labeled as asthmatic. Older males more often were given the diagnosis of emphysema, whereas older females were more readily labeled as having asthma or chronic bronchitis.

The confusion was also illustrated by a recently published survey [9] in which 121 respondents from 11 countries of Europe and North America were asked how they would label 4 different model patients in corresponding with colleagues. It was most prominent in the labeling of the disease condition of a 68-year-old male patient, lifelong cigarette smoker with productive morning cough, poorly reversible severe airway obstruction and altered arterial blood gases, but no clinical signs of emphysema; his diagnosis was given no less than 31 names by these respondents. The survey also stressed the indiscriminate use of the term 'chronic bronchitis', since 9% of the respondents used it without qualifying labels in this patient. The same unqualified term was used by 46% in a model patient with chronic mucus hypersecretion without airway obstruction, by 8% in an obstructed, mildly allergic patient with a previous history of asthma, and by 3% in a patient with radiological and functional signs of emphysema. Aside from the confusion generated by the term, this clearly illustrates the poor precision conferred by the term in describing the individual patient.

Surprisingly, however, when the respondents were asked to indicate whether they found the term 'chronic bronchitis' referred to a well-defined clinical entity, on average 79% of the respondents answered positively. This percentage was lowest among the Finnish (58%) and highest among the Italian (100%) chest physicians, responding to the survey. When it was asked *how frequently* the term was used to refer to individual patients in communicating with other physicians, 68% of the respondents reported that they used the term either 'often' or 'always'. Again there were differences between countries, since all the USA chest physicians reported this frequent use and only 58% of the Spanish physicians. Most other terms referring to airway obstruction, like COPD, CAO (chronic airway obstruction), CAL (chronic airflow limitation) or 'chronic obstructive bronchitis' were considered less well defined and were also used less often.

The conclusion of this international survey clearly is that, despite a bias in the sample towards older and more university-based chest physicians, many of these respondents were confused about the use of the term 'chronic bronchitis', but were either unaware of it or did not care!

Is There Justification for The Use of 'Chronic Bronchitis'?

As any other term in '-itis', bronchitis implies inflammation, here of the bronchial wall. Such inflammation is present in acute bronchitis due to infection. In many patients with chronic bronchitis and hypersecretion, infection is absent. The presence and the role of inflammation in the central airways has been subject to controversy. Earlier studies had indicated the absence of inflammatory cells in stable chronic bronchitis. However, a later study [10] more clearly demonstrated that inflammation is present in cartilaginous airways of patients satisfying MRC criteria for chronic bronchitis and that it even provided a better morphological indication for it than mucus gland hypertrophy. In patients whose mucus hypersecretion persisted after cessation of smoking, inflammation was still marked in central as well as peripheral airways, whereas there was least inflammation in ex-smokers without mucus hypersecretion [11]. Some criticisms have been raised on the methods of scoring inflammation in these studies [12]; one of these is that inflammatory cells were mostly lymphocytes and mononuclear cells and not polymorphonuclear (PMN) cells. This contrasts with findings during acute infectious episodes where central airways become crowded with PMN cells. Although additional studies seem to be required to settle this issue, the presence of at least some inflammation seems to justify the use of the term 'bronchitis' in chronic mucus hypersecretion.

However, inflammation was detected to an even larger extent in the peripheral airways of smokers with airway obstruction [13]. Even in asthma, the presence of inflammation with predominant eosinophils has prompted experts [14] to propose the term 'chronic eosinophilic bronchitis' to characterize this condition. Inflammation thus appears to be a feature of all forms of obstructive and hypersecretory airway disease; hence, its lack of specificity does not seem very helpful in differentiating the various disease entities, especially in the absence of histological studies that are quite difficult to perform in a clinical setting. In defining disease entities, it should be preferable to use more easily accessible clinical criteria and to take into account the prognostic significance of such criteria.

Which Terminology Should Be Used?

In many patients with clinical features of hypersecretion, the concomitant presence of persistent obstruction can also be demonstrated. Hypersecretion within central airways and airway obstruction in peripheral airways were found to be two largely independent phenomena, with prognosis for morbidity and mortality mostly dependent on the latter, while prognosis of hypersecretion in itself is generally considered good [5]. In view of this, it seems preferable to use the term 'chronic obstructive lung disease' (COLD) when hypersecretion and obstruction are combined, because it refers to both obstruction as the most important feature and to a disease affecting the lung.

One could also in this situation consider using the term 'chronic obstructive bronchitis', although it proved to be less popular in the recent international survey [9]. However, if obstruction is present without hypersecretion – a frequent occurrence in ex-smokers – the use of the term 'chronic bronchitis' would then be quite confusing, in view of the earlier MRC definitions. If hypersecretion is present in patients with chronic airway obstruction, one may obviously like to indicate this by adding, as qualifying labels, either 'with mucus hypersecretion' or 'with chronic bronchitis'. Both terms should also be considered in patients with hypersecretion without obstruction. Given the confusion generated by 'chronic bronchitis', preference should be given to indicating the presence of mucus hypersecretion directly through the use of this term.

Conclusions

A quite precise clinical definition was given to the term 'chronic bronchitis' in the early sixties to refer to the presence of chronic mucus hypersecretion. In view of recent histological findings of widespread bronchial inflammation, the term could find justification. However, I feel that recommending further extensive use of the term to refer to all patients with nonasthmatic, nonemphysematous obstructive airway disease would greatly add to the present confusion. Hence, the term does not need redefinition from the orignal MRC proposals, but it could be appropriately replaced by 'mucus hypersecretion'. To characterize the disease with predominant and persistent airway obstruction, COPD or COLD are the preferred terms.

Acknowledgement

The author is grateful to Dr. Neil Pride (London) for many stimulating discussions on the appropriate use of terminology in obstructive lung diseases.

References

1 Ciba Guest Symposium: Terminology, definitions and classifications of chronic pulmonary emphysema and related conditions. Thorax 1959;14:286–299.
2 American Thoracic Society: Definitions and classification of chronic bronchitis, asthma, and pulmonary emphysema. Am Rev Respir Dis 1962;85:762–768.

3 Medical Research Council: Definition and classification of chronic bronchitis for clinical and epidemiological purposes. Lancet 1965;i:775–779.
4 Thurlbeck W: Aspects of chronic airflow obstruction. Chest 1977;72:341–349.
5 Peto R, Speizer F, Cochrane A, Moore F, Fletcher C, Tinker C, Higgins I, Gray R, Richards S, Gilliland J, Norman-Smith B: The relevance in adults of air-flow obstruction, but not of mucus hypersecretion, to mortality from chronic lung disease. Am Rev Respir Dis 1983;128:491–500.
6 Fletcher C, Pride N: Definitions of emphysema, chronic bronchitis, asthma, and airflow obstruction: 25 years on from the Ciba Symposium. Thorax 1984;89:81–85.
7 Orie N, Sluiter H, de Vries K, Tammeling G: Chronische aspecifieke respiratoire aandoeningen. Ned Tijschr Geneeskd 1961;105:2136–2139.
8 Dodge R, Cline M, Burrows B: Comparisons of asthma, emphysema, and chronic bronchitis diagnoses in a general population sample. Am Rev Respir Dis 1986;133:981–986.
9 Pride N, Vermeire P, Allegra L: Diagnostic labels in chronic airflow obstruction: Responses to a questionnaire with model case histories in North American and Western European countries. Eur Respir J 1989;2:702–709.
10 Mullen B, Wright J, Wiggs B, Pare P, Hogg J: Reassessment of inflammation of airways in chronic bronchitis. Br Med J 1985; 291:1235–1239.
11 Mullen B, Wright J, Wiggs B, Pare P, Hogg J: Structure of central airways in current smokers and ex-smokers with and without mucus hypersecretion: Relationship to lung function. Thorax 1987;42:843–848.
12 McCusker K, Hoidal J: Leukocyte function and chronic bronchitis. Semin Respir Infect 1988;3:5–13.
13 Cosio M, Hale KA, Niewohner DE: Morphologic and morphometric effects of prolonged cigarette smoking on the small airways. Am Rev Respir Dis 1980;22:265–271.
14 Barnes P: A new approach to the treatment of asthma. N Engl J Med 1989;321:1517–1527.

Prof. P. Vermeire
Department Geneeskunde
Universiteit Antwerpen (UIA)
Universiteitsplein, 1
B–2610 Antwerpen-Wilrijk (Belgium)

Respiration 1991;58(suppl 1):10–12

0025–7931/91/0587–0010 $ 2.75/0

Risk Factors for Chronic Bronchitis and Chronic Obstructive Lung Disease

Gérard Huchon

Université René-Descartes, Hôpital Ambroise-Paré, Boulogne, France

Key Words. Chronic bronchitis · Chronic obstructive lung disease · Tobacco smoke · α_1-Antitrypsin · Epidemiology

Abstract. Among the risk factors for chronic bronchitis and chronic obstructive lung disease, only smoking and α_1-antitrypsin deficiency effects have been well demonstrated. Other factors, as air pollution, occupational exposure and childhood lung diseases may have an influence, but on a lower scale. The prevention of chronic bronchitis and chronic obstructive lung disease remains mainly based on antismoking programs.

The traditional concept regarding the origins of chronic obstructive lung diseases following exposure to smoking is that they result from the inhalation of cigarette smoke responsible for mucous hypersecretion, which in turn induces recurring bronchial infections leading to chronic bronchitis and obstructive lung disease. This concept was challenged in 1977 by Fletcher and Peto [1]. Inhalation of cigarette smoke, they suggested, gives rise to two different lung diseases. One is due to hypertrophy of mucous glands responsible for mucous hypersecretion and recurring bronchial infections. The other is an airway disease with emphysema, leading up to airflow limitation and respiratory failure. Both conditions differ in regard to susceptibility to cigarette smoke – which accounts to 50% for hypertrophy of mucous glands, and to 10–15% for airway obstruction – and in regard to the effect of smoking cessation, which brings mucous hypersecretion to a stop and prevents all further excessive aggravation, whilst it does not afford integral restoration of the airways in case of obstruction. Besides smoking, only one other risk factor for chronic obstructive lung disease could be demonstrated. This is not the case, however, for other potential risk factors, as indicated in table 1 [2].

Effects of Cigarette Smoke

The effects of smoking on the airways are the best and most documented item. An inverse relation between cigarette consumption and expiratory flow was shown in a given population [3]. But a significant number of patients, in spite of being active smokers, show no lung function abnormality. Figure 1 shows the possible effects of smoking on lung function in smokers susceptible to the effects of cigarette smoke, as well as in smokers who were not sensitive to cigarette smoke [1]. In the patients who smoked and were susceptible to the effects of cigarette smoke, smoking cessation slowed down the speed of pulmonary function deterioration to that of the nonsmokers, but did not normalize the lung function.

Any other risk factors are difficult to establish because of the mildness of their effects compared to those of smoking.

α_1-Antitrypsin Deficiency

There is highly serious evidence proving the effects of α_1-antitrypsin deficit on the protease-antiprotease imbalance. Among the possible effects of such a deficit is the occurrence of emphysema of the pan-lobular type. Conversely, there have been few studies on the physiological consequences of such a deficit for the lung and on how it affects the survival of patients with this condition. Nonetheless, it was shown that subjects with PiZZ-type phenotype have a lower probability of survival than normal subjects and that this survival is even lower in smokers with α_1-antitrypsin deficit [4].

Table 1. Risk factors for chronic obstructive lung disease [2]

Demonstrated		Putative
Agent	Cigarette smoke	Air pollution
		Occupational pollution
		Passive smoking
		Virus
		Socio-economic status
		Alcohol
Host	α_1-Antitrypsin deficiency	Age
		Gender
		Genetic
		Airway hyperresponsiveness

Table 2. Age-adjusted risk factors for obstructive airways disease [13]

Documented	Not documented
Airflow limitation	Drinking habits
Smoking habits	Social class
Chronic bronchitis	Physical measurements
Respiratory symptoms	Genetic markers
History of infections	
Familial respiratory diesease	

A population of men and women, aged 16–74 years, in the town of Tecumseh was studied from 1962 to 1979.

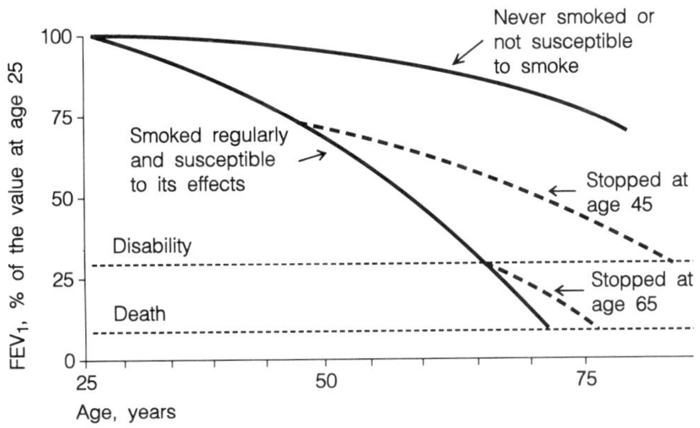

Fig. 1. Risks for various male smokers [1]. The differences between the lines illustrate the effects that smoking and smoking cessation can have on the forced expiratory volume/second (FEV_1) of a smoker who is at risk of developing chronic obstructive lung disease.

Air Pollution

Many cross-sectional studies suggest that air pollution, whatever its nature is, can be responsible for respiratory symptoms and reduced lung function. Thus, a survey conducted in the area of Los Angeles compared the importance and nature of air pollution with lung function [5]. The town of Lancaster was considered a clean area as opposed to Burbank, known for its pollution due to oxidants, and to the town of Long Beach, characterized by the presence of petrochemical plants causing pollution due to particles, hydrocarbons and sulfur dioxide. The percentage of patients with airflows <75% of the predicted value was significantly higher in the polluted areas of Burbank and Long Beach than in the Lancaster area.

Another survey, which proved more rewarding as it was longitudinal, was conducted over a 9-year period by Lend et al. [6] in the Netherlands. They compared the expiratory flows of subjects in two areas: a rural area free from air pollution, Vlagtwedde, and another area, Vlaardingen, which was polluted by refineries releasing sulfur monoxide and smokes. They were able to demonstrate that the mean reduction in vital capacity and the mean expiratory flow in milliliters per year, following adjustment for smoking habits, was higher in the polluted than in the nonpolluted area.

Occupational Exposure

In a longitudinal study conducted over a period of 12 years by Kauffmann et al. [7] in 575 men aged 30–54 years and working in the Paris area, evidence for the effects of occupational exposure to mineral or organic dusts on the lung function was shown. The yearly reduction of forced expiratory volume/second was significantly higher, by 10–20 ml per year, in the subjects exposed to occupational air pollutants, whatever their smoking level was.

Childhood Lung Diseases

There are retrospective and longitudinal studies suggesting that childhood illnesses may be responsible for respiratory diseases in adults [8, 9]. The prevalence of lung involvement was shown to be higher in subjects with parents who had sustained respiratory tract infections in their childhood. The mother's smoking also seems to increase the prevalence of respiratory symptoms [10]. Retrospective studies suggested that pediatric lung diseases account for an important risk factor of obstructive disease developing in adulthood, whether the patients were smokers or not [11].

Social Status

Various studies, British in particular, focused on the possible role of social class on the occurrence of obstructive lung disease. It was observed that mortality from lung disease increased quite significantly in underprivileged classes [12]. But this was demonstrated to be probably due to smoking, as lower classes are known to smoke more.

Predictor

The studies conducted aimed at predicting the probability of chronic obstructive lung disease on the basis of certain risk factors. The reference study is that of Higgins et al. [13]. They studied a population of men and women aged 16–74 years in the town of Tecumseh from 1962 to 1979 and were able to show that certain factors did not significantly influence the occurrence of chronic obstructive lung disease, whilst others had a very clear effect (table 2). Among the risk factors, a reduction in expiratory flow in the subjects sensitive to the effects of tobacco smoke on the respiratory tract suggests that it is possible to detect in which smokers a reduction will occur at a certain level of exposure to smoking, which would have no effect in other subjects not susceptible to the effects of smoking. This shows a way to detect subjects who are sensitive to the effects of cigarette smoke. The most important risk factors were age, daily cigarette consumption, possible alteration of smoking habits and the observed value of forced expiratory volume/second.

Prevention

One cannot talk about chronic obstructive lung diseases without mentioning prevention. Prevention rests on antismoking programs, attempts to produce less toxic cigarettes, and air pollution control whether outdoors or indoors. It also includes the prevention of childhood respiratory diseases and, finally, early detection of obstructive pulmonary diseases in order to avoid subsequent breakdown in patients susceptible to tobacco smoke.

References

1 Fletcher C, Peto R: The natural history of chronic airflow obstruction. Br Med J [Clin Res] 1977;i:1645–1658.
2 Buist AS: Smoking and other risk factors; in Murray JF, Nadel J (eds): Textbook of Respiratory Medicine. Philadelphia, Saunders, 1988, vol 42, pp 1001–1029.
3 Burrow B, Knudson RJ, Chine MG, Lebowitz MD: Quantitative relationships between cigarette smoking and ventilatory function. Am Rev Respir Dis 1977;115:195–205.
4 Larsson C: Natural history and life expectancy in severe $alpha_1$-antitrypsin deficiency, PiZ. Acta Med Scand 1978;204: 345–351.
5 Rokaw SN, Detels R, Coulson AH, Sayre JW, Tashkin DP, Allwright SS, Massey FJ: The UCLA population studies of chronic obstructive respiratory disease. Chest 1980;78:252–262.
6 Lend RV, Kok TJ, Peset Reig R, Quanjer PH, Schouten JP, Orie NGM: Decreases in VC and FEV with time: Indicators for effects of smoking and air pollution. Bull Eur Physiopathol Respir 1981;17:775–792.
7 Kauffmann F, Drouet D, Lelouch J, Brille D: Twelve years spirometric changes among Paris area workers. Int J Epidemiol 1979;8:201–212.
8 Schenker MB, Samet JM, Speizer FE: Risk factors for childhood respiratory disease. Am Rev Respir Dis 1983;128: 1038–1043.
9 Tager I, Speizer FE: Role of infection in chronic bronchitis. N Engl J Med 1975;13:563–571.
10 Ware JH, Dockery W, Spiro A, Speizer FE, Ferris BG: Passive smoking, gas cooking, and respiratory health of children living in six cities. Am Rev Respir Dis 1984;129:366–374.
11 Burrows B, Knudson RJ, Lebowitz MD: The relationship of childhood respiratory illness to adult obstructive airway disease. Am Rev Respir Dis 1977;115:751–760.
12 Holland WW: Chronic obstructive lung disease prevention. Br J Dis Chest 1988;82:32–44.
13 Higgins MW, Keller JB, Becker M, Howatt W, Landis JR, Rotman H, Weg JG, Higgins I: An index of risk for obstructive airways disease. Am Rev Respir Dis 1982;125:144–151.

Prof. Gérard Huchon
Université René-Descartes
Hôpital Ambroise-Paré
9, avenue Charles-de-Gaulle
F-92104 Boulogne Cedex (France)

Respiration 1991;58(suppl 1):13–17

0025–7931/91/0587–0013 $ 2.75/0

Bronchoalveolar Clearance

Demetri Pavia

Department of Thoracic Medicine, The Royal Free Hospital and School of Medicine, London, UK

Key Words. Alveolar clearance · Cough · Lung permeability · Mucociliary clearance · Mucus

Abstract. The lungs possess several mechanisms for cleansing themselves from locally produced biological debris and inhaled, deposited soluble and insoluble materials. Insoluble particles deposited on the conducting, ciliated airways will be primarily removed by mucociliary clearance, over a period of several hours, with cough acting as a back-up clearance mechanism. Insoluble particles deposited in the non-ciliated, alveolated regions of the lungs will be cleared primarily by the macrophages very slowly, with a biological half-life of several months. Soluble substances can pass through paracellular pathways and be cleared via the blood stream.

Introduction

Airborne particles can enter the lungs either via the nose or the mouth during inspiration. Those particles which deposit in the lungs will be subsequently cleared by mechanism(s) depending upon their initial site of deposition. In this way the lungs can keep themselves clean and sterile even when exposed to a polluted atmosphere. Soluble particles will enter the blood stream and will be predominantly cleared from the lungs by this route. Insoluble particles deposited in the conducting airways will be cleared primarily by mucociliary transport with cough as a back-up clearance mechanism. Insoluble particles deposited in the alveolated regions will be removed by the scavenging action of the alveolar macrophages [1–3].

Clearance from the Alveolated Regions of the Lungs

Particles deposited in the respiratory (alveolated) regions of the lungs are cleared by two main processes: absorptive and non-absorptive.

Absorptive Process

Hydrophilic substances which are not transported through the cell can nevertheless pass through the epithelium by passive diffusion through the junctions, i.e. the paracellular pathway. For hydrophilic solutes in the molecular weight range of 50–100,000 Da, the permeability of the vascular epithelium is approximately 10 times greater than that of the alveolar epithelium. The 'effective' pore radius of the endothelium is 4–8 nm whereas that of the alveolar epithelium is of the order of 1 nm.

An index of the rate at which small-molecule solutes leak from the lungs into the circulating blood can be derived by measuring the rate of disappearance of radioactivity from the lungs, using a gamma camera positioned over the chest, following the inhalation of aerosolised ^{99m}Tc diethylenetriamine pentacetic acid (^{99m}Tc-DTPA) (fig. 1). The molecular weight of DTPA is 492 Da and it has a molecular radius of 0.6 nm. Because of the recirculation of 'leaked' radioactivity in the blood, there is a need to correct the disappearance of lung radioactivity for blood background. Such a correction can be achieved by

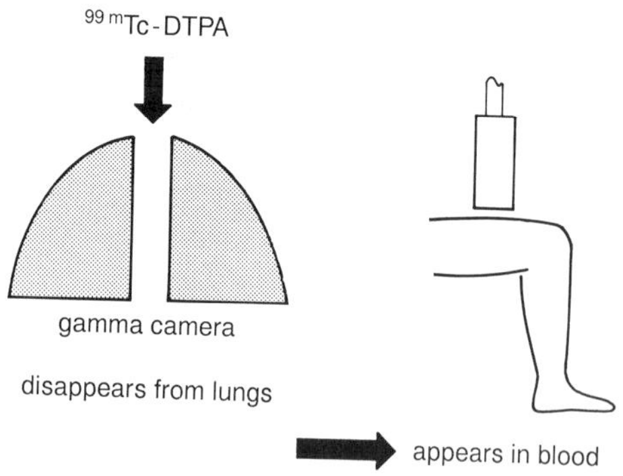

Fig. 1. Schematic diagram of the technique used for measuring lung permeability. Inhaled, deposited ^{99m}Tc-DTPA aerosol in the lungs is removed via the blood stream. By courtesy from Dr. J.E. Agnew.

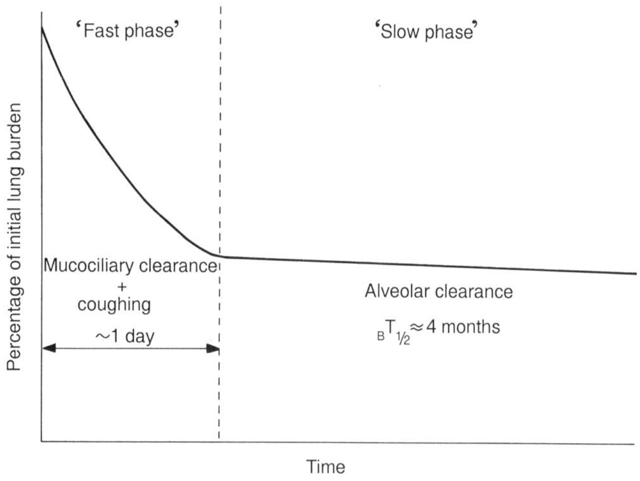

Fig. 2. Schematic diagram of the retention/clearance of inhaled insoluble particles from the human lungs.

recording the presence of radioactivity over a suitable vascular site, e.g. thigh (using a separate scintillation detector) or by carefully selecting a region of interest within the gamma camera (used for monitoring lung radioactivity) field of view [4]. The disappearance of lung radioactivity is followed for say 15–30 min after which period of time an intravenous bolus of ^{99m}Tc-DTPA (a calibration dose) is administered. The ensuing increase in count rate over the lung region relative to that over the vascular region gives a factor by which the blood background can be estimated and subsequently subtracted from the 'lung + blood' clearance curve. From the corrected clearance curve, the half-time (the time taken for the radioactivity to be reduced by one half) can be calculated for ^{99m}Tc-DTPA to pass from the lungs to the blood. The 'epithelial barrier' becomes more permeable in many disease processes. This suggests that abnormal epithelial function allows albumin, with a molecular weight of 65,000 Da (radius: about 4 nm), to leak into the alveolar space.

Non-Absorptive Process

The alveolar macrophage is largely responsible for the removal of particles from the non-ciliated, respiratory regions of the lungs [5-6]. Alveolar macrophages have a diameter of about 15–50 μm and lie in contact with surfactant (lipoprotein material) which lines the alveoli. Inhaled particles which have been phagocytosed by macrophages are transported from the non-ciliated air spaces to the ciliated airways and subsequently removed from the lungs via the mucociliary clearance mechanism. The transport of the macrophages from the alveolated regions to the ciliated airways may depend on the difference in surface tension between the two regions. The surfactant fluid has a lower surface tension than the bronchial fluid which may induce the former to spread into the conducting airways carrying with it the macrophages. The gradient in the interfacial surface tension between the two regions is enhanced during each inspiration and this may enhance macrophage transport from the alveolated regions. Alternatively, macrophages containing phagocytosed particles may migrate through the epithelial wall into the interstitial spaces, and then (1) deposit the particles for distribution in the lymphatics, (2) re-enter the ciliated airways and/or (3) deposit the particles around peribronchial or perivascular locations – places of long-term 'storage'.

The number of ingested particles has been found to be proportional to the size of the particles. Particles 2–3 μm in diameter are optimally phagocytosed, whereas particles less than 0.3 μm have been shown to be only minimally taken up by the macrophages. Another factor that plays a role in the phagocytosis of particles is their chemical composition.

Insoluble particles deposited in the alveoli are cleared very slowly with a biological half-time of the order of 3–4 months (fig. 2). Clearance from the alveoli is often represented by a multi-exponential curve which is attributed to different clearance mechanisms. The fastest exponential, with a half-time of days/weeks, is thought to be due to alveolar macrophage activity. A slower phase, with a half-time of several months, is thought to represent slow penetration through the alveolar epithelium and dissolution of the particles.

Clearance from the Conducting Airways of the Lungs

Clearance of inhaled deposited particles from the conducting airways (i.e. from the level of the terminal bronchioles to the trachea) of the lungs takes place mainly by two clearance mechanisms namely mucociliary transport [7-10] and cough [11-13]. The combination of these two clearance mechanisms gives rise to what is often termed tracheobronchial clearance. These two clearance mechanisms will be considered further in terms of two experiments which were carried out in our laboratory.

The diagnosis of Kartagener's syndrome relies on a clearly defined triad: dextrocardia, chronic sinusitis and bronchiectasis. Patients with this syndrome when adequately investigated have been shown to have ciliary dyskinesia and/or immotility together with a variety of underlying ultrastructural abnormalities including missing dyneim arms, essential for the bending action of the cilia. As a result of this, it is not surprising that lung mucociliary clearance has been reported to be very severely impaired or absent in these patients [14-15].

We have investigated the lung mucociliary clearance in a group of 8 patients in whom Kartagener's triad had not been established in so far as they lacked proof of bronchiectasis with one exception, but who nevertheless had dextrocardia accompanied by bronchial and sinus sepsis [16]. Lung mucociliary clearance was measured using an objective, non-invasive radioaerosol technique. Polystyrene particles, firmly labelled with the radionuclide ^{99m}Tc ($T_{½}$ = 6 h), were inhaled by the patients and their subsequent clearance from the lungs by mucus transport was monitored with suitably collimated scintillation counters positioned over the patients' chests. The tracheobronchial clearance for these patients was compared with that for a group of 34 healthy subjects with similar physical characteristics, tobacco consumption and initial topographical distribution of the tracer particles in the lungs as those for the patients. Tracheobronchial clearance was found to be statistically significantly reduced in the patients compared to the healthy control group (fig. 3). This in itself is not surprising. What is of interest, however, is how relatively 'good' the tracheobronchial clearance for the patients was, since previous studies carried out over shorter observation periods concluded that lung mucociliary clearance was virtually absent in patients with primary ciliary dyskinesia syndrome (patients with/without dextrocardia but having sinusitis and bronchiectasis and ciliary abnormalities).

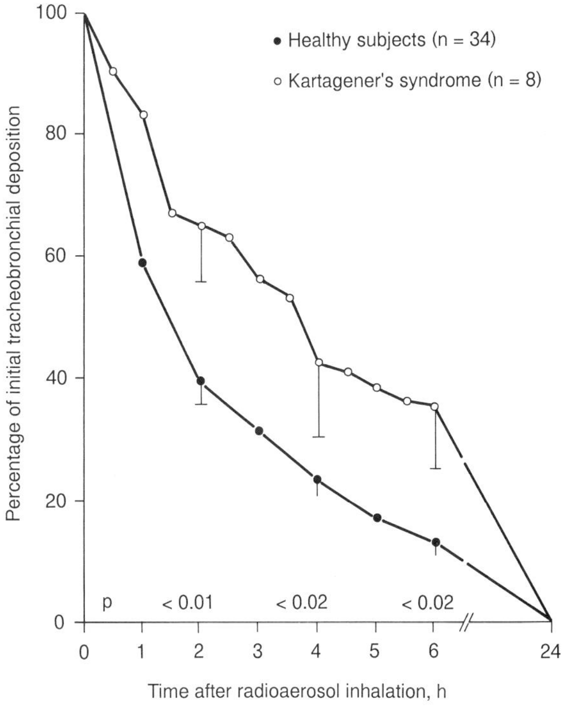

Fig. 3. Mean ± SEM tracheobronchial retention curves for 8 patients with Kartagener's syndrome and 34 'matched' healthy subjects. Adapted from Pavia et al. [16].

One possibility for this 'apparent' good tracheobronchial clearance in the patients might be that the back-up clearance mechanism, cough, played a major role in clearing the radioaerosol from the lungs. Cough is a reserve mechanism which comes into action in emergency situations in health such as after the inhalation of a foreign substance and in lung disease (e.g. asthma, chronic bronchitis) where mucociliary transport is impaired [7]. However, theory suggests that the high linear air velocities that are necessary for shearing the mucus from the bronchial walls and expel it from the lungs cannot be attained beyond the 8th-10th airway generations of the human lung (Weibel's model) [12]. The role played by cough in the tracheobronchial clearance of our patients with dextrocardia was examined by ensuring that all sputum samples during the 6-hour observation period were collected and their radioactive content measured. When this radioactive content was 'added back' to the tracheobronchial clearance curve for the patients a 'sputum-corrected' tracheobronchial clearance curve was generated. Despite this correction, tracheobronchial clearance was still 'relatively good' although the clearance now resembled the lung mucociliary clearance seen in patients with chronic bronchitis with a mean age double that of our patients and who had smoked some 30 cigarettes daily for some 50 years. The possibility, of course, existed that our patients with dextrocardia swallowed some sputum during coughing. As a check for this, a plot of number of coughs versus time of observation (i.e. 6 h) of tracheobronchial clearance showed 0 correlation whereas if swallowing played a major role then a positive (significant) correlation would have been expected.

If lung mucociliary clearance is as bad in patients with primary ciliary dyskinesia syndrome as it has been suggested, it is difficult to see how these patients are able to remove their secretions from the 16th airway generation (terminal bronchioles, i.e. foot of mucociliary escalator) to the 10th, or thereabouts, airway generation where cough is said to be effective. In order to explain this, one will have to propose that cough is effective in clearing lung secretions throughout all the ciliated airways in the presence of excess secretions, as indeed one in vitro study has suggested [17]. An alternative explanation might be that other mechanism(s) might be operating in our lungs helping to clear secretions cephalad.

It is well known that patients with global respiratory muscle weakness are prone to hypoventilation and respiratory failure [18]. If the expiratory muscles are involved in a significant way then it is possible that such patients may have impaired cough efficiency and theoretically such patients could develop chest infections unless satisfactory physiotherapy is provided. It is of interest to note that patients with diaphragmatic muscle weakness are also considered to be susceptible to respiratory tract infections even though expiratory muscle strength in such patients is normal. The second experiment which we carried out was to investigate the tracheobronchial clearance of patients with respiratory muscle weakness affecting only the diaphragm.

The tracheobronchial clearance of 7 patients with symptoms of bilateral diaphragmatic muscle weakness was compared with that of a control healthy group of similar physical characteristics, smoking habits and initial topographical distribution of the tracer radioaerosol within their lungs [19]. The mean $\pm$SD area under the tracheobronchial clearance curve for these patients ($262 \pm 80\% \cdot h$) was found to be statistically significantly larger ($p < 0.02$) than that for the control group ($142 \pm 41\% \cdot h$). This indicated that the patients with bilateral diaphragmatic muscle weakness had a reduced tracheobronchial clearance compared to the healthy controls. The patients did not cough or expectorate any sputum voluntarily during the 6-hour observation period for tracheobronchial clearance nor at the end of this period when they were instructed to cough vigorously.

If tracheobronchial clearance is reduced in patients with bilateral diaphragmatic weakness and cough is not a complicating factor, then it must be concluded that it is due to a reduction attributable to either impairment of mucociliary transport or some other clearance mechanism(s).

It is of interest to note that it has previously been reported that healthy subjects and patients with chronic bronchitis are capable of increasing their tracheobronchial clearance in response to vigorous exercise, such as briskly cycling on a bicycle ergometer for say half an hour. This increase was attributed, by the investigators, to either (a) mechanical effect of increased lung movement or (b) an effect of the autonomic nervous system mediated via the parasympathetic pathway producing stimulation of airway glands and/or sympathetic stimulation of cilia owing to exercise-induced catecholamine release.

The combination of our evidence of a reduced tracheobronchial clearance in patients with bilateral diaphragmatic weakness and the converse, that is an enhancement in clearance in healthy subjects and chronic bronchitics during vigorous exercise, lends support to the anecdotal reports of a clearance mechanism operating in the lungs – sometimes referred to as 'milking' or 'squeezing' of the lungs – during mechanical movement thereby encouraging the flow of airway secretions cephalad. If this is so then one can start visualising the situation whereby in patients with primary ciliary dyskinesia syndrome (in whom mucociliary transport is said to be absent) that such a 'milking' or 'squeezing' of the airways during normal breathing in conjunction with the two-phase (air-airway secretions interaction) can 'push' secretions from the distal parts of lungs to the proximal airways where their clearance by cough can be achieved. Such a theory might well account for the longevity of such patients although it does not answer why the same is not true for patients with cystic fibrosis who, nevertheless, have grossly abnormal mucus.

References

1 Green GM: Alveobronchiolar transport mechanisms. Arch Intern Med 1973;131:109–114.
2 Morrow PE: Alveolar clearance of aerosols. Arch Intern Med 1973;131:101–108.
3 Lauweryns JM: Alveolar clearance and the role of the pulmonary lymphatics. Am Rev Respir Dis 1977;115:625–683.
4 Jones JG, Minty BD, Royston D: The physiology of leaky lungs. Br J Anaesth 1982;54:705–721.
5 Bailey MR, Fry FA, James A: The long-term clearance kinetics of insoluble particles from the human lung. Ann Occup Hyg 1982;26:273–290.
6 Jones JG: Clearance of inhaled particles from the alveoli: in Clarke SW, Pavia D (eds) Aerosols and the Lung, Clinical and Experimental Aspects. London, Butterworths, 1984, pp 170–196.
7 Pavia D: Lung mucociliary clearance; in Clarke SW, Pavia D (eds) Aerosols and the lung: Clinical and Experimental Aspects. London, Butterworths, 1984, pp 127–155.
8 Camner P: Clearance of particles from the human tracheobronchial tree. Clin Sci 1980;59:79–84.
9 Wanner A: Clinical aspects of mucociliary transport. Am Rev Respir Dis 1977;116:73–125.
10 Yeates DB, Gerrity TR, Garrard CS: Particle deposition and clearance in the bronchial tree. Ann Biomed Eng 1981;9: 577–592.
11 Clarke SW: The role of two-phase flow in bronchial clearance. Bull Physio Pathol Respir 1973;9:359–372.
12 Leith DE: Cough. Phys Ther 1968;48:439–447.
13 Sutton PP: Chest physiotherapy and cough; in Clarke SW, Pavia D (eds) Aerosols and the Lung: Clinical and Experimental Aspects. London, Butterworths, 1984, pp 156–169.
14 Mossberg B, Afzelius BA, Elliasson R, Camner P: On the pathogenesis of obstructive lung disease. A study on the immotile-cilia syndrome. Scand J Respir Dis 1978;59:55–65.
15 Rossman CM, Forrset JB, Lee RMKW, Newhouse MT: The dyskinetic cilia syndrome. Ciliary motility in immotile cilia syndrome. Chest 1980;78:580–582.
16 Pavia D, Agnew JE, Sutton PP, Lopez-Vidriero MT, Currie DC, Cole PJ, Clarke SW: Impaired mucus clearance in patients with chronic bronchial sepsis, sinusitis and dextrocardia. Respiration 1988;53:187–196.
17 Scherer PW: Mucus transport by cough. Chest 1981;80:830–833.
18 Newsom-Davis J, Goldman M, Loh L: Diaphragm function and alveolar hypoventilation. Q J Med 1976;45:87–100.
19 Mier A, Laroche C, Agnew JE, Vora H, Clarke SW, Green M, Pavia D: Tracheobronchial clearance in patients with bilateral diaphragmatic weakness. Presented at the SEPCR Meet, Athens, 1988.

Dr. Demetri Pavia, MSc, PhD, CPhys, FIPSM, FInstP
Boehringer Ingelheim Limited
Ellesfield Avenue
Bracknell
Berkshire, RG12 4YS (UK)

Respiration 1991;58(suppl 1):18–21

0025–7931/91/0587–0018 $ 2.75/0

Late Asthmatic Reactions, Airway Inflammation and Chronic Asthma in Toluene-Diisocyanate-Sensitized Subjects[1]

Leonardo M. Fabbri, Marina Saetta, Guido Picotti, Christine E. Mapp

Interuniversity Center on Cellular and Molecular Mechanisms of Lung Injury, Universities of Brescia, Genova, Milan, Padova and Parma, Italy

Key Words. Asthma · Occupational diseases · Airway obstruction · Bronchial provocation tests · Epithelium

Abstract. To determine the importance of airway inflammation for exacerbation and prognosis of asthma induced by toluene diisocyanate (TDI), we first examined sensitized subjects during asthmatic reactions induced by exposure to TDI in the laboratory. We observed that late and dual, but not early, asthmatic reactions induced by TDI are accompanied by a transient increase of airway responsiveness, bronchoalveolar neutrophilia followed by eosinophilia and by an increase of LTB4 and albumin in bronchoalveolar lavage fluid. All these effects were prevented by pretreatment with prednisone. In addition, we examined the lung pathology of 1 sensitized subject who died after exposure at work. The pathologic features of fatal asthma induced by TDI and of chronic asthma induced by TDI suggest the importance of inflammation for the exacerbation and prognosis of the disease.

Introduction

Sensitized subjects may develop symptoms of asthma after exposure to isocyanates at their place of work [1, 2]. After challenges with isocyanates in the laboratory, sensitized subjects develop immediate, late and dual asthmatic reactions [3]. Dual and late asthmatic reactions are more frequent than the early ones [4], and like allergen-induced dual and late asthmatic reactions, they have probably more relevance to the natural history of asthma than the immediate asthmatic reactions. In fact, late asthmatic reactions are usually more severe, last longer, respond to steroids but not to bronchodilators, are more resistant to therapy, and subjects sensitized to toluene diisocyanate (TDI) who develop dual or late asthmatic reactions continue to have asthma upon cessation of exposure [5]. Longitudinal studies suggest that the majority of subjects with occupational asthma remain asthmatic months and years after the cessation of exposure. The mechanisms of late asthmatic reaction and persistence of asthma after cessation of exposure are unknown.

We speculated that TDI might cause late asthmatic reactions and increase bronchial responsiveness by causing an acute inflammatory reaction in the airways, and that airway inflammation may be responsible for the persistence of occupational asthma induced by isocyanates.

Asthmatic Reactions, Airway Hyperresponsiveness and Airway Inflammation Induced by TDI

To test these hypotheses, we examined sensitized subjects during asthmatic reactions induced by exposure to TDI in the laboratory. We observed that late and dual, but not early, asthmatic reactions are asso-

[1] Supported in part by the Italian National Research Council, grants No. 87.00266.56 and 87.01476.04, a grant from the European Community for Coal and Steel, and a special grant from Regione Veneto.

ciated with a transient increase of bronchial responsiveness [6] and, at the same time, with an increase of neutrophils followed by eosinophils [7], and of LTB4 [8] and albumin [7] in bronchoalveolar lavage fluid. All these effects could be prevented by pretreatment with prednisone [9], but not with the nonsteroidal anti-inflammatory agent indomethacin [10]. Aerosolized steroids alone, e.g. beclomethasone [11, 12], dexamethasone isonicotinate [13], or combined with salbutamol [14] completely inhibit late asthmatic reactions induced by TDI, whereas theophylline [11] has a partial, verapamil [11], ketotifen [15], salbutamol alone [14], atropine [16] and cromolyn [11] have no protective effect.

All these studies, taken together, support the hypothesis that in the late and dual, but no in the early, asthmatic reaction induced by TDI, bronchoconstriction and airway inflammation are involved, and that polymorphonuclear leukocytes are required for hyperresponsiveness to occur. Although one of the inflammatory mediators (i.e. LTB4) was measured during late asthmatic reactions induced by TDI, the identification of the structure and source of all chemotactic factors which attract neutrophils and eosinophils in the airspaces, and the identification of the mediators released by these cells remain to be established.

Pathology of TDI Asthma

Only one report is available on documented occupational asthma death induced by a low exposure to isocyanate at work in a subject previously demonstrated to be sensitized to TDI [17]. Lung pathology included some characteristic features almost invariably reported in status asthmaticus and some findings different from previous reports on nonoccupational asthma. Macroscopically, the lungs appeared overinflated and did not collapse on opening of the pleural cavities. The airways were plugged with mucus containing abundant exudate. Microscopy showed morphological abnormalities of both airways and lung parenchyma. In the airways, extensive epithelial desquamation, edema of the bronchial wall, diffuse infiltration of inflammatory cells including eosinophils and neutrophils and marked thickening of the basement membrane were observed in addition to the almost pathognomonic presence of extensive plugging of the bronchioles. The mucous glands were hyperplastic, and the bronchial smooth muscle was hypertrophic and disarrayed with loss of the usual regular intersections of fibers that criss-cross each other unevenly and form whirls.

While hypertrophy of airway smooth muscle was almost invariably present in previous reports on nonoccupational asthma, the disarray of smooth muscle fibers had not been described before. Abnormal in vitro responsiveness of the airway smooth muscle after exposure to isocyanates was reported in an animal model [18]. In addition, a contractile effect of TDI on smooth muscle from different sources has recently been demonstrated in vitro, and it seems to be mediated by the release of tachykinins [C.E. Mapp, pers. comm.]. Although McKay and Brooks' [18] study did not include a morphologic description of the tissue, the disarray of smooth muscle fibers observed in asthma death due to isocyanates suggests that this chemical may directly affect airway smooth muscle.

Morphologic abnormalities were present not only at the bronchial level, but also within the alveolar walls. Areas of acute emphysema alternated with focal areas of atelectasis. The presence of acute emphysema was confirmed by the observation of destroyed alveolar wall which appeared as fragments of septa floating in the alveolar spaces. These areas of focal destruction were adjacent to areas of perfectly intact alveolar walls. Interestingly, these focal lesions have not been described in nonoccupational asthma and are very similar to the parenchymal abnormalities observed in the early stage of emphysema in a group of smokers in whom the classic indices of emphysema were still normal [19, 20]. This observation needs to be verified with more complete studies, since some investigators have recently described a possible role of loss of elastic recoil in the pathogenesis of asthma [21]. The elastic loads against which bronchial smooth muscle contracts are important determinants of the degree of airway narrowing, and alveolar wall destruction, together with bronchial wall edema, may facilitate airway narrowing by decreasing these elastic loads.

Acute alveolitis may develop in subjects sensitized to methyldiphenyl-diisocyanate after a specific inhalation challenge [22]. Polymorphonuclear infiltration of the alveolar walls is present in asthma death due to isocyanates, thus suggesting that, at variance with asthma death induced by allergens, death induced by isocyanates in sensitized subjects may be associated with parenchymal injury.

Asthmatic Reactions and Prognosis of TDI-Induced Asthma

Among the pathologic features observed in the airways, eosinophilic infiltration of the mucosa and submucosa was particularly pronounced [17]. Interestingly, Paggiaro et al. [23] reported that subjects with persistent asthma after cessation of exposure have chronic inflammation of the airway mucosa, characterized by slight infiltration of eosinophils. Indeed, longitudinal studies suggest that the majority of subjects with occupational asthma continue to have persistent asthma months and years after the cessation of exposure [24]. We have recently completed a follow-up study [25] on 35 subjects with different types of reaction to the inhalation challenge and observed that the few subjects who recovered, in addition to being younger and having a shorter duration of exposure and disease, developed either early or dual asthmatic reactions at the screening inhalation challenge with TDI, whereas none of the subjects who continued to be exposed and/or developed a late asthmatic reaction at presentation recovered completely. The subjects with dual asthmatic reactions who recovered had a milder reaction compared to those who had dual asthmatic reactions at presentation and did not recover.

Whether the recovery (or failure to recover) is related to the degree of airway inflammation remains to be established, but the results of our study combined with the results of several other studies strongly suggest that this might be the case. Interestingly, in all longitudinal studies published so far, subjects who continued to be exposed, even if at presumably lower concentrations of isocyanates or other sensitizing agents, were those who did not recover from occupational asthma.

Acknowledgment

We sincerely thank the subjects who contributed to these studies. We also acknowledge the technical assistance of Luigi Zedda and Stefano Miante and thank Licia Tolin and Susan Lees for reviewing and editing the manuscript.

References

1 Fabbri LM, Salvaggio JE (eds): Occupational asthma. Folia Allergol Immunol Clin 1985;32:1–65.
2 Chan-Yeung M: Occupational asthma update. Chest 1988;93:407–411.
3 Pepys J, Hutchroft BJ: Bronchial provocation tests in etiologic diagnosis and analysis of asthma. Am Rev Respir Dis 1975;112:829–859.
4 Mapp CE, Boschetto P, Dal Vecchio L, Maestrelli P, Fabbri LM: Occupational asthma due to isocyanates. Eur Respir J 1988;1:273–279.
5 O'Byrne PM, Dolovich J, Hargreave FE: Late asthmatic responses. Am Rev Respir Dis 1987;136:740–751.
6 Mapp CE, Polato R, Maestrelli P, Hendrick DJ, Fabbri LM: Time course of the increase in airway responsiveness associated with late asthmatic reactions to toluene diisocyanate in sensitized subjects. J Allergy Clin Immunol 1985;75:568–572.
7 Fabbri LM, Boschetto P, Zocca E, Milani GF, Pivirotto F, Burlina A, Plebani M, Licata B, Mapp CE: Bronchoalveolar neutrophilia during late asthmatic reactions induced by toluene diisocyanate (TDI). Am Rev Respir Dis 1987;136:36–42.
8 Zocca E, Boschetto P, Mapp CE, Milani GF, Pivirotto F, Fabbri LM: LTB4-like substance in bronchoalveolar lavage supernatant released during asthmatic reactions induced by toluene diisocyanate in sensitized subjects. J Appl Physiol, in press.
9 Boschetto P, Fabbri LM, Zocca E, Milani GF, Pivirotto F, Dal Vecchio A, Plebani M, Mapp CE: Prednisone inhibits late asthmatic reactions and airway inflammation induced by toluene diisocyanate in sensitized subjects. J Allergy Clin Immunol 1987;80:261–267.
10 Fabbri LM, Di Giacomo R, Dal Vecchio L, Zocca E, De Marzo N, Maestrelli P, Mapp CE: Prednisone, indomethacin and airway responsiveness in toluene-diisocyanate-sensitized subjects. Bull Eur Physiopathol Respir 1985;21:421–426.
11 Mapp CE, Boschetto P, Dal Vecchio L, Crescioli S, De Marzo N, Paleari D, Fabbri LM: Protective effect of antiasthma drugs on late asthmatic reaction and increased responsiveness induced by toluene diisocyanate in sensitized subjects. Am Rev Respir Dis 1987;136:1403–1407.
12 De Marzo N, Fabbri LM, Crescioli S, Plebani M, Testi R, Mapp CE: Dose-dependent inhibitory effect of inhaled beclomethasone on late asthmatic reactions and increased airway responsiveness to methacholine induced by toluene diisocyanate in sensitized subjects. Pulmonary Pharmacol 1988;1:15–20.
13 Tossin L, Leproux GB, De Marzo N, Crescioli S, Mapp CE, Fabbri LM: Dosauxison inhibits late asthmatic reactions induced by toluene diisocyanate in sensitized subjects. Ann Allergy, in press.
14 Moscato G, Gherson G, Dellabianca A, et al: Salbutamol plus beclomethasone inhibits early and late asthmatic reactions to toluene diisocyanate (TDI) whereas salbutamol alone inhibits neither (abstract). Eur Respir J 1989;2(suppl 5):398.
15 Paggiaro PL, Bacci E, Talini D, Dente FL, Rossi O, Pulera N, Fabbri LM, Giuntini C: Atropine does not inhibit late asthmatic responses induced by toluene diisocyanate in sensitized subjects. Am Rev Respir Dis 1987;136:1237–1241.
16 Tossin L, De Marzo N, Crescioli S, Mapp CE, Fabbri LM: Ketotifen does not inhibit asthmatic reactions induced by toluene diisocyanate in sensitized subjects. Clin Exp Allergy 1989;19:177–182.
17 Fabbri LM, Danieli D, Crescioli S, Bevilacqua P, Meli S, Saetta M, Mapp CE: Fatal asthma in a toluene-diisocyanate-sensitized subject. Am Rev Respir Dis 1988;137:1494–1498.

18 McKay RT, Brooks SM: Hyperreactive airway smooth muscle responsiveness after inhalation of toluene diisocyanate vapors. Am Rev Respir Dis 1984;129:296-300.

19 Saetta M, Shiner RJ, Angus GE, Kim WD, Wang NS, King M, Ghezzo N, Cosio MG: Destructive index: A measurement of lung parenchymal destruction in smokers. Am Rev Resp Dis 1985;131:764-768.

20 Saetta M, Ghezzo H, Kim WD, et al: Loss of alveolar attachments in smokers. A morphometric correlate of lung function impairment. Am Rev Respir Dis 1985;132:894-900.

21 Moreno RH, Hogg JC, Pare PD: Mechanics of airway narrowing. Am Rev Respir Dis 1986;133:1171-1180.

22 Mapp CE, Dal Vecchio L, Boschetto P, Fabbri LM: Combined asthma and alveolitis due to diphenylmethane diisocyanate (MDI) with demonstration of no crossed respiratory reactivity to toluene diisocyanate (TDI). Ann Allergy 1985;54:424-429.

23 Paggiaro PL, Paoletti P, Bacci E, et al: Eosinophils in bronchoalveolar lavage (BAL) of patients with toluene diisocyanate (TDI) asthma after cessation of work. Am Rev Respir Dis 1987;135:A234.

24 Paggiaro PL, Bacci E, Talini FL, Giuntini C: Prognosis of occupational asthma induced by isocyanates. Bull Eur Physiopathol Respir 1987;23:583-586.

25 Mapp CE, Chiesura Corona P, De Marzo N, Fabbri LM: Persistent asthma due to isocyanates. Am Rev Respir Dis 1988; 137:1326-1329.

Leonardo M. Fabbri, MD
Istituto di Medicina del Lavoro
Università di Padova
Via J. Facciolati 71
I-35127 Padova (Italy)

Respiration 1991;58(suppl 1):22–29

0025–7931/91/0587–0022 $ 2.75/0

Transplantation for End-Stage Lung Disease

George Cremona, Tim Higenbottam, John Wallwork

Department of Respiratory Physiology, Papworth Hospital, Cambridge, UK

Key Words. Lung transplantation · Heart-lung transplantation · Lung rejection · Obliterative bronchiolitis

Abstract. The last decade has seen lung and heart-lung transplantation move from experimental procedures to clinical treatments. Innovative surgical techniques combined with the use of ciclosporin as an immunosuppressive agent have enabled successful transplantation in a wide range of end-stage lung diseases. Exclusion criteria for selecting recipients have relaxed, and improved preservation techniques have facilitated distant donor organ procurement and decreased peri-operative mortality. A range of techniques for the physiological monitoring of the graft as well as diagnosis of major complications such as rejection and opportunistic infection have been introduced. Obliterative bronchiolitis remains a major challenge to the immunologist and to the chest physician in terms of etiology, pathogenesis and treatment. As survival rates improve with improved management, lung and heart-lung transplantations are contributing towards effective treatment of end-stage pulmonary disease as well as providing new insight into pulmonary physiology and into mechanisms of lung disease.

Introduction

Transplantation of the lungs in patients with end-stage pulmonary disease has now become a valid therapeutic option in spite of a discouraging early history. The first human lung transplantation was performed in 1963 on a patient with cancer of the left lung and chronic obstructive airways disease [1]. The patient died after only 18 days. Combined heart-lung transplantation (HLT) was first performed in humans by Cooley et al. [2] in 1968 in a 2-month-old child with Eisenmenger syndrome. The patient only survived for 14 h after implantation due to respiratory failure. Early attempts were beset by problems and it was only until a number of significant improvements were made in various aspects of transplantation that clinical transplantation of the lungs became possible.

Two developments have made the most significant contribution to successful lung transplantation. The introduction of ciclosporin [3], which acts by blocking the production of interleukin-2 and inhibiting the function of the T-helper lymphocyte [4], reduced the requirement for steroids and consequently minimized the risk of poor wound healing especially of the airway anastomosis. Secondly the development in primates by Reitz et al. [5] of the technique of transplanting heart and lungs en bloc achieved better anastomotic healing apparently by conserving an intact mediastinal collateral circulation from the coronary arteries to the lower trachea. Successful HLT in humans was first undertaken in 1981 [6] in a patient with primary pulmonary hypertension. The problem of airway ischaemia in unilateral lung transplantation was resolved by bronchial omentopexy [7] which enables satisfactory revascularization of the bronchial mucosa. A successful single-lung transplantation (SLT) with long-term survival was performed in 1983 [8]. Combined with the substitution of high-dose corticosteroid with ciclosporin [9], this technique has been successfully extended to the transplantation of both lungs [10] in 1986 and although concern remains regarding anastomotic healing, recent reports [11] have been quite encouraging. These advances together with improved organ preservation techniques [12] and more stringent criteria for recipient selection [13] have contributed to successful transplant programmes in various centres in both North America and Europe.

Pre-Operative Management

Assessment of Patients for Transplantation

Transplantation of the lungs has been limited to relatively small numbers of patients due to the paucity of suitable donors. For this reason this treatment has been offered only to those patients with end-stage lung disease who have the best potential for long-term survival with a capacity for full rehabilitation. With the availability of three procedures of lung transplantation, careful tailoring of the transplantation procedure for the individual and specific disease has developed to ensure maximal benefit to the patient as well as maximal use of the donor organs. All transplantation centres have developed intensive pre-transplantation assessment programmes that apply fairly stringent selection criteria.

Indications for Heart-Lung Transplantation

Initially HLT was established as a method for treating severe primary or secondary pulmonary vascular disease [6]. This technique has since been effectively extended to a wide range of chronic end-stage lung diseases [14] (table 1). The patients with parenchymal lung disease and good cardiac function may themselves become heart donors in what has become known as the domino procedure [15]. This is especially effective if the domino heart is placed in a patient with increased right ventricular afterload as the likelihood of post-operative acute right heart failure is probably reduced.

A wide variety of chronic lung diseases have been treated successfully by HLT. These have included emphysema, pulmonary fibrosis, bronchiectasis, sarcoidosis, α_1-antitrypsin deficiency and histiocytosis X. One of the major developments has been the extension of this procedure to treat patients with cystic fibrosis which in our own series has become the largest single disease group., Interestingly, these patients were not initially considered suitable for transplantation because of concerns regarding sepsis in the immunosuppressed transplanted cystic fibrosis patient and the possible recurrence of the inherited defect in the transplanted organs. However, they have been shown to survive HLT with excellent lung function [16] and the epithelial abnormality has not recurred when measured using mucosal potential difference [17].

Table 1. Indications for lung transplantation

	HLT	SLT	DLT
End-stage fibrotic lung disease			
Cryptogenic fibrosing alveolitis	+	+	
Extrinsic allergic alveolitis	+	+	
Sarcoidosis	+	+	
Pneumoconiosis	+	+	
Scleroderma	+	+	
Chronic obstructive lung disease			
Emphysema	+	+	+
α_1-Antitrypsin deficiency	+	+	+
Bronchiolitis obliterans	+	+	+
Pulmonary sepsis			
Cystic fibrosis	+		+
Bronchiectasis	+		+
Pulmonary hypertension			
Primary pulmonary hypertension	+	+[1]	
Eisenmenger syndrome	+		
Chronic pulmonary thromboembolic disease	+		
Pulmonary parenchymal disease with separate cardiac dysfunction	+		
Miscellaneous			
Lymphangioleiomyomatosis	+		
Eosinophilic granuloma	+		

[1] With reversible right ventricular function.

Indications for Single-Lung Transplantation

The ideal indication for SLT is fibrotic disease [8]. With this procedure, the compliant transplanted lung with low vascular resistance receives preferential ventilation and perfusion. This has in fact been demonstrated by serial ventilation-perfusion radioisotope scanning. In patients with increased compliance such as emphysema or increased vascular resistance such as primary pulmonary hypertension an imbalance in ventilation perfusion ratio was expected to occur. However, a number of SLT in such patients have been undertaken and Mal et al. [18] have reported the ventilation-perfusion (V/Q) data post-SLT in 2 patients with emphysema. Although the patients continued to

Table 2. Recipient selection criteria

Life expectancy < 18 months
Pulmonary hypertension
Mixed venous oxigen saturation < 63%
Cardiac index < 1.5 litres · min^{-1} · m^{-2}
Parenchymal lung disease
FEV_1 < 30% predicted
Evidence of cor pulmonale
Hypoxic hypercapnic respiratory failure
Age
< 50 years - heart-lung
< 50 years - double lung
< 60 years - single lung
No high-dose steroid therapy
Absence of non-reversible organ dysfunction
No previous major thoracic surgery (HLT/DLT)
Psycho-social stability

Table 3. Donor criteria

Age below 40 years
No major thoracic trauma
Normal chest radiograph
Absence of infected sputum
Absence of systemic infection
Normal lung compliance: peak inspiratory pressure < 2.7 kPa
Normal gas exchange: arterial partial pressure of oxygen > 15 kPa with fractional inspired oxygen < 30%
Minimal inotropic requirements (dopamine or dobutamine < 10 μg · kg^{-1} · min^{-1})
Normal electrocardiogram

Table 4. Immunosuppression for lung and heart-lung transplantation

Preoperative	
Ciclosporin	4–6 mg/kg p.o. 4 h before anaesthetic induction
Azathioprine	2–3 mg/kg as above
Methylprednisolone	1,000 mg i.v.
Postoperative	
Ciclosporin	6–10 mg/kg/day p.o. adjusted to renal function to maintain serum levels between 150–400 ng/ml
Azathioprine	2–2.5 mg/kg/day adjusted to white cell count ≦4,500
Rejection	
Methylprednisolone	0.5 g i.v. for 3 days
Prednisolone [1]	10 mg/day until resolution

[1] Some centres use a maintenance dose of 0.2 mg/kg/day prednisolone.

have airway obstruction evidenced by spirometry, there was no V/Q mismatch. However, all these patients have been transplanted recently and the long-term outcome remains to be seen.

Currently, sepsis in the recipient is an absolute contra-indication to SLT.

Indications for Double-Lung Transplantation

Double-lung transplantation (DLT) potentially offers advantages over HLT such as permitting 2 patients to benefit from a single donor and avoiding concurrent as well as asynchronous rejection of the heart and the accelerated coronary artery disease associated with it. Currently, DLT is mainly performed on patients with chronic obstructive lung disease such as emphysema and bilateral septic conditions such as cystic fibrosis and bronchiectasis. However, DLT carries a high peri-operative mortality rate and there is still a need for advances in the surgical technique [10].

Criteria for Recipient Selection

Patients considered suitable for transplantation are placed on the active waiting list when their life expectancy is less than 18 months. Selection criteria for these patients include declining lung function and lack of response to steroid therapy [19], a forced expiratory volume in 1 s (FEV_1) below 30% predicted, suggesting advanced disease [20]; hypoxic hypercapnic respiratory failure and the development of cor pulmonale have also been identified as indicators of a poor prognosis [21] (table 2). In our centre we have used the 12-min walk test [22] tolerance. A 12-min walking distance less than 500 m with a drop in arterial oxygen saturation below 60% indicates severe impairment. Exclusion criteria have narrowed as experience with these procedures has increased. The presence of other organ damage is a contra-indication for transplantation, although candidates with concurrent liver disease have been considered for HLT and liver transplantation [23]. Aspergilloma, previous pleurectomy and pleurodesis [13] in HLT and DLT continue to be exclusion criteria. Relative contra-indications include steroid dependence, presence of *Aspergillus fumigatus* in the sputum and insulin-dependent diabetes mellitus.

Criteria for Donor Selection

Lung and HLT is limited by the availability of donor organs. The mechanical ventilation necessary after brain death exposes the lungs to a variety of possible injuries which, like infection, atelectasis and neurogenic pulmonary oedema, may preclude them from being used for transplantation. Direct major chest trauma is also a contra-indication to donation (table 3). The current accepted criteria include age below 40 years, normal chest radiograph, normal electrocardiogram, adequate gas exchange, absence of pulmonary or systemic infections, and minimal inotropic dependence. These strict criteria severely limit the number of organs accepted for donation; only 10–15% of the suitable heart donors are actually also accepted as lung donors.

Size is also important as donor organs too large for the recipient thorax can result in atelectasis and intrapulmonary shunting. Once accepted, potential recipients are matched for size using donor and recipient chest radiographs. The most important index in this regard appears to be the thoracic vertebral height. Serological matching for cytomegalovirus (CMV) between donor and recipient is also performed as CMV pneumonitis may follow the transplantation of organs from a CMV-positive donor to a CMV-negative recipient leading to CMV pneumonitis [24, 25].

Early transplantation programmes were severely limited by the lack of adequate graft preservation which necessitated that donor and recipient operations be carried out in adjoining theatres. This problem has now been overcome by various means of organ preservation techniques. Cardiopulmonary bypass with whole body cooling [26, 19] and autoperfusion of the heart-lung block [27] have been successfully used by various groups. An extremely simple and effective method is the hypothermic pulmonary artery flush with a blood-based solution after intravenous infusion of prostacyclin to dilate the pulmonary vascular bed [28]. This method requires little additional equipment or personnel, and excellent graft preservation has been achieved with ischaemic times of up to 4 h [12].

Post-Operative Management

Other than immunosuppression and a vigorous control of fluid balance, early post-transplantation care is similar to that following routine cardiac surgery. Efforts are made for the early extubation and subsequent mobilization of the patient as the denervated lung is not responsive to secretions below the tracheal anastomosis. There is a transitory deterioration in lung function coinciding with radiological signs of interstitial oedema [29]. The genesis of this disorder is probably due to various causes such as graft ischaemia during preservation, surgical trauma; relative fluid overload as well as a lack of lymphatic drainage. Fluids are initially restricted and diuretics administered to achieve a negative fluid balance within the second post-operative day. These measures limit the fluid accumulation which occurs in the first few days.

Immunosuppression

Immunosuppressive therapy in lung and HLT is based on ciclosporin, azathioprine and, in the immediate post-operative period, antithymocyte globulin (table 4). This allows flexibility in ciclosporin dosage and is particularly useful in those patients with post-operative renal problems. In most centres, especially in North America, steroids in the form of prednisone are introduced 14–21 days following transplantation. In our centre, however, the use of steroids is reserved for rejection episodes. During the first month after transplantation, intravenous methyl prednisolone is used, and after this time oral prednisolone is administered, a short course of 1 mg/kg/day, tapered to 10 mg/day until resolution.

Rejection

Probably the most important problem in the management of lung transplantation patients is the early diagnosis of lung rejection and distinguishing it from opportunistic lung infection. On purely clinical grounds, this has been found to be impossible [30, 31], as both conditions can present with pyrexia, dyspnoea and cough and comparable physical signs of both crackles and wheezes [32]. Radiological findings are also non-specific and in early rejection may even be normal [33].

Transbronchial Lung Biopsy

Initially, endomyocardial biopsy [34, 35] was routinely used to monitor rejection in the lung in HLT patients. This technique is now considered unsatisfactory as pulmonary rejection may occur in the absence [14, 36, 37] or asynchronously [38] with cardiac rejection. Moreover this technique is obviously unsuitable in SLT and DLT. We have therefore stopped using routine endomyocardial biopsy [39] and adopted transbronchial lung biopsy as a means for obtaining tissue [32]. Using the larger alligator forceps, 3–4 biopsies up to 5 mm in size are taken from the upper, middle (or lingula on the left) and lower lobe. The principal morphological changes in acute rejection [40] are those of a circumscribed perivascular lymphocytic infiltrate which may later extend to the intra-alveolar septa and even into the alveoli themselves. This is clearly distinguishable from the changes due to opportunistic infection where perivascular oedema, without a dense cellular component is more typical. Intra-alveolar exudates are common together with pathognomonic features of infection. In the diagnosis of acute lung rejection, transbronchial lung biopsy has a sensitivity of 70% and a specificity of 100% [41].

Pulmonary Function Monitoring

Dynamic lung volumes decrease significantly during most episodes of rejection and/or infection. This change in function improves following appropriate therapy. Other indices also vary in these conditions but are not suitable for diagnosis due to the increased measurement error [42]. Domiciliary spirometric measurement is a non-invasive procedure and can be performed on a daily basis. Patients are issued with pocket-battery-operated spirometers which measure the forced expiratory volume in 1 s (FEV_1) and the forced vital capacity (FVC). Variations as small as 5% on 2 consecutive days are sufficient for the patients to refer themselves to the hospitals for biopsy [43]. Although these measurements are not specific, they are very sensitive and allow close monitoring of the physiological function of the graft.

Infection

Infection is one of the leading causes of morbidity and mortality in lung transplant or HLT recipients [24, 44]. In our first 66 patients, 9 deaths were attributable to fatal infections. Practically any pathogen can cause infection in these immunocompromised patients [45], and there is a definite tendency for these organisms to invade the transplanted lung. In the early post-operative phase, bacteria are the most frequent cause of pneumonia, gram-negative rods and *Staphylococcus aureus* being the most common pathogens. In our series, 3 patients died of bacterial pneumonia.

CMV infection is most common 4–8 weeks post-operatively. CMV pneumonia was the cause of death in 4 of our patients. Three of these deaths occurred before our donor-recipient serologic CMV matching policy (see above) was put into force. During that time out of 17 patients, mismatching occurred on 7 occasions and 6 of these patients developed primary CMV infection. Five infections affected the lung and 1 the gastro-intestinal tract. Three of these patients died [25]. Following the adoption of donor-recipient matching, there have been only 2 instances of primary CMV pneumonia, 1 of which followed the use of infected blood. However, in 11 cases of reactivation of CMV all these patients had sustained 1 episode of rejection requiring augmentation of immunosuppressive therapy prior to the appearance of the infection.

There is a significant temporal overlap between CMV pneumonia and early rejection of the lung. The two conditions can produce a very similar clinical picture and a similar profile of cell types in bronchoalveolar lavage. A problem exists in diagnosing CMV infection; the presence of nuclear inclusion bodies on cells prepared for routine cytologic analysis is very specific but not very sensitive, on the other hand methods such as the detection of viral antigens [46] in broncho-alveolar lavage cells are very sensitive but not very specific to CMV pneumonia.

Intravenous ganciclovir has been shown to be effective in the treatment of CMV pneumonia [47]. We institute therapy at the outset of infection either on the basis of a threefold increase in antigenic titres, or on the basis of biopsy results. Ganciclovir is also used prophylactically in high-risk patients (mismatched, or patients with previous CMV infection) in conditions requiring augmented immunosuppression.

Herpes simplex (HSV) infection in solid-organ transplants nearly always occurs as a reactivation in recipients who had HSV before transplantation or acquired it from the environment. HSV pneumonia occurred in 7 of our patients, all of whom had positive serology prior to transplantation and all developed mucocutaneous lesions before the onset of pneumonia. These episodes were associated with augmented immunosuppression and previous CMV infection. Due to these observations we have adopted a policy of prophylactically treating patients who are HSV positive prior to surgery with oral acyclovir for 3 months following transplantation.

Pneumocystis carinii pneumonia is also frequently encountered in lung transplantation patients [24]. Diagnosis is usually established by demonstrating the presence of the organisms in lavage fluid or bioptic material. Prophylaxis with oral cotrimoxazole (480 mg b.i.d.) is effective in reducing this problem [48].

Immunosuppressed transplant recipients are at risk from any type of fungus. Invasive aspergillosis carries a particularly grave prognosis and occurs predominantly in allografts of profoundly immunosuppressed recipients or in patients having already suffered CMV infection. Diagnosis is histological requiring transbronchial lung biopsy or broncho-alveolar lavage. The specimens are stained with Grocott's silver stain which demonstrates the fungal hyphae. Intravenous amphotericin B in full therapeutic doses is useful in treating this infection but only following a prolonged course to achieve a total dose of 1.2–1.5 g over 2–3 months. This treatment is unfortunately associated with some degree of irreversible renal impairment and does not reverse the decline in lung function caused by the infection.

Obliterative Bronchiolitis

Obliterative bronchiolitis is defined as an inflammatory disorder of the small airways leading to the obstruction and destruction of pulmonary bronchioles. First reported in 1984 [49], it has now been widely reported affecting between 10–54% of long-term HLT survivors [50]. It has also been described although less commonly for SLT recipients but not in DLT. Whether this is due to the lower numbers of patients undergoing SLT and DLT, or whether this is due to the lower antigenic load as is claimed by those in favour of the latter procedures is a question that will only be resolved with time and greater numbers.

The etiology and pathogenesis of obliterative bronchiolitis are as yet unknown, but various hypotheses have been put forward which include chronic or repeated episodes of rejection [51], infections, especially viral, which tend to activate the cellular immune system causing the reappearance of alloreactive lymphocytes, or a combination of the two leading to peripheral airway injury.

HLT has provided the most extensive experience of long-term allograft function. There is a strong correlation between evidence of fibrotic changes on biopsy and failure of the recipients to achieve satisfactory lung volume after transplantation. The major factor associated with fibrosis within the biopsy is the frequency of rejection. Among these patients a number proceed to develop irreversible airflow obstruction despite repeated courses of augmented immunosuppression. A maintenance immunosuppression utilizing ciclosporin A, prednisolone and azathioprine seems to be more effective than earlier regimens utilizing only ciclosporin and prednisolone. Constant lung function monitoring and close histological surveillance for early evidence of fibrosis and consequently repeated pulse steroids until lung function returns to expected values, has lowered the mortality and morbidity at our centre and elsewhere. Once pulmonary function begins to progressively decline there is as yet no known treatment to reverse or even impede this process.

Long-Term Prospects for Lung Transplantation

Long-term survival following HLT, SLT and DLT are comparable at 60–70% actuarial survival rates at 2 years although numbers for the latter two procedures are still relatively low. Slight differences reflect patients selection rather than any true differences in procedure. HLT and DLT survivors generally achieve normal spirometry, slightly reduced gas transfer. SLT patients transplanted for end-stage fibrotic lung disease retain a persistent restrictive pattern and a reduced gas transfer.

On the whole, lung transplant patients seem to fall into three broad categories. Around a half of them have minimal problems with optimal immunosuppressive regimens. Another group seem to suffer from repeated rejection episodes soon after transplantation which necessitate the addition of continuous low-dose oral steroids to the standard immunosuppressive regimen. These patients are more likely to achieve suboptimal lung function but are quite stable and lead high-quality lives. A third group, which may stem from the preceding one, go on to irreversible deterioration of graft function. It is for this group that efforts are required to identify with greater precision the risk factors involved and to develop new immunosuppressive therapy perhaps even to the graft pre-operatively to reduce subsequent rejection.

References

1 Hardy JD, Webb WR, Dalton ML, et al: Lung homotransplantation in man. JAMA 1963;186:1065–1074.
2 Cooley DA, Bloodwell RD, Hallman GL, et al: Organ transplantation for advanced cardiopulmonary disease. Ann Thorac Surg 1969;8:30.
3 Calne RY, White DJG, Thiru S, et al: Cyclosporin A in patients receiving renal allografts from cadaver donors. Lancet 1978;ii: 1323–1327.

4 Kahan BD: Drug therapy: Cyclosporin. N Engl J Med 1989; 321:1725–1738.
5 Reitz BA, Burton NA, Jamieson SW, et al: Heart and lung transplantation, autotransplantation, and allotransplantation in primates with extended survival. J Thorac Cardiovasc Surg 1980;80:360–372.
6 Reitz BA, Wallwork J, Hunt SA, et al: Heart-lung transplantation: Successful therapy for patients with pulmonary vascular disease. N Engl J Med 1982;306:557–564.
7 Lima O, Goldberg M, Peters WJ, et al: Bronchial omentopexy in canine lung transplantation. J Thorac Cardiovasc Surg 1982; 83:418–421.
8 Toronto Lung Transplant Group: Unilateral lung transplantation for pulmonary fibrosis. N Engl J Med 1986;314:1140–1145.
9 Goldberg M, Lima O, Morgan E, et al: A comparison between cyclosporin A and methylprednisolone plus azathioprine on bronchial healing following canine autotransplantation. J Thorac Cardiovasc Surg 1983;85:821–826.
10 Cooper JD, Patterson GA, Grossman R, et al: Double-lung transplant for advanced chronic obstructive lung disease. Am Rev Respir Dis 1989;139:303–307.
11 Noiclerc M: Double lung transplantation for cystic fibrosis (abstract). Annu N Am Cystic Fibrosis Conf, October 1989.
12 Hakim M, Higenbottam TW, Bethune D, et al: Selection and procurement of combined heart and lung grafts for transplantation. J Thorac Cardiovasc Surg 1988;95:474–479.
13 Harjula A, Baldwin JC, Oyer PE, et al: Recipient selection for heart-lung transplantation. Scand J Thorac Cardiovasc Surg 1988;22:193–196.
14 Penketh A, Higenbottam TW, Hakim M, et al: Heart and lung transplantation in patients with end-stage lung disease. Br Med J 1987;295:311–314.
15 Cavarocchi NC, Badellino M: Heart/heart-lung transplantation. The domino procedure. Ann Thorac Surg 1989;48:130–133.
16 Scott JP, Higenbottam TW, Hutter JA, et al: Heart-lung transplantation for cystic fibrosis. Lancet 1988;ii:192–194.
17 Wood AM, Higenbottam TW, Jackson M, et al: Airway mucosal bioelectric potential differences in cystic fibrosis after lung transplantation. Am Rev Respir Dis 1989;140:1645–1649.
18 Mal H, Andreassian B, Pamela F, et al: Unilateral lung transplantation in end-stage pulmonary emphysema. Am Rev Respir Dis 1989;140:797–802.
19 Turner-Warwick M, Borrows B, Johnson A: Crytptogenic fibrosing alveolitis: Response to corticosteroid treatment and its effect on survival. Thorax 1980;35:593–599.
20 Bishop JM, Cross KW: Physiological variables and mortality in patients with various categories of chronic respiratory disease. Bull Eur Physiopathol Respir 1984;20:495–500.
21 Siassi B, Moss AJ, Dooley RR: Clinical recognition of cor pulmonale in cystic fibrosis. J Pediatr 1971;78:794–805.
22 McGavin CR, Artininti M, Nave H, et al: Dyspnoea, disability and distance walked: Comparison of estimates of exercise performance in respiratory disease. Br Med J 1978;2:241–244.
23 Wallwork J, Williams R, Calne RY: Transplantation of liver, heart and lungs for primary biliary cirrhosis and primary pulmonary hypertension. Lancet 1987;ii:182–184.
24 Dummer JS, Montero CG, Griffith BP, et al: Infections in heart-lung transplant recipients. Transplantation 1986;41:725–729.
25 Hutter JA, Scott JP, Wreghitt T, et al: The importance of cytomegalovirus in heart-lung transplant recipients. Chest 1989; 95:627–629.
26 Baumgartner WA, Williams GW: Cardiopulmonary bypass with profound hypothermia. An optimal preservation method for multiorgan procurement. Transplantation 1989;47:123–127.
27 Hardesty RL, Griffith BP: Autoperfusion of the heart and lungs for preservation during distant procurement. J Thorac Cardiovasc Surg 1987;87:11.
28 Wallwork J, Jones K, Cavarocchi N, et al: Distant procurement of organs for clinical heart-lung transplantation using a single flush technique. Transplantation 1987;44:654–658.
29 Chiles C, Guthaner PF, Jamieson SW, et al: Heart-lung transplantation: The post-operative chest radiograph. Radiology 1985;154:299.
30 Penketh ARL, Higenbottam TW, Hutter JA, et al: Clinical experience in the management of pulmonary opportunistic infection and rejection in recipients of heart-lung transplants. Thorax 1988;43:762–769.
31 McGregor CGA, Jamieson SW: Clinical heart and lung transplantation. Br Med J 1985;290:1682.
32 Higenbottam TW, Stewart S, Penketh A, et al: Transbronchial lung biopsy for the diagnosis of rejection in heart-lung transplant patients. Transplantation 1988;46:532–539.
33 Millet B, Higenbottam TW, Flower CDR, et al: The radiographic appearances of infection and acute rejection of the lung after heart-lung transplantation. Am Rev Respir Dis 1989; 140:62–67.
34 Reitz BA, Gaudinani VA, Hunt SA, et al: Diagnosis and treatment of allograft rejection in heart-lung transplant recipients. J Thorac Cardiovasc Surg 1983;85:354–361.
35 Caves PK, Stinson EB, Graham AF, et al: Percutaneous transvenous endomyocardial biopsy. JAMA 1973;225:288–291.
36 Cooper DTC, Novitzky D, Rose AG, et al: Acute pulmonary rejection precedes cardiac rejection following heart-lung transplantation in a primate model. J Heart Transplant 1986;5: 29–32.
37 McGregor CGA, Baldwin JC, Jamieson SW, et al: Isolated pulmonary rejection after combined heart-lung transplantation. J Thorac Cardiovasc Surg 1985;90:623–626.
38 Griffith BP, Hardesty RL, Trento A, et al: Asynchronous rejection of heart and lungs following cardiopulmonary transplantation. Ann Surg 1985;40:488.
39 Higenbottam TW, Hutter JA, Stewart S, et al: Transbronchial biopsy has eliminated the need for endomyocardial biopsy in heart-lung recipients. J Heart Transplant 1988;7:435–439.
40 Hutter JA, Stewart S, Higenbottam TW, et al: Histologic changes in heart-lung transplant recipients during rejection episodes and at routine biopsy. J Heart Transplant 1988;7: 440–444.
41 Sadeghi AM, Guthaner DF, Wexler L, et al: Healing and revascularization of the tracheal anastomosis following heart-lung transplantation. Surg Forum 1982;33:236–238.
42 Otulana BA, Higenbottam TW, Scott JP, et al: Lung function associated with histologically diagnosed acute lung refection and pulmonary injection in heart-lung transplant patients. Am Rev Respir Dis 1990;141:329–332.
43 Otulana BA, Higenbottam TW, Ferrari L, et al: The use of home spirometry in detecting acute lung rejection and infection following heart-lung transplantation. Chest 1990;97:353–357.

44 Brooks RG, Hofflin JM, Jamieson SW, et al: Infectious complications in heart-lung transplant recipients. Am J Med 1985; 79:412–422.
45 Hill RB, Rowlands IT, Rifkind D: Infectious pulmonary disease in patients receiving immunosuppressive therapy for organ transplantation. N Engl J Med 1964;271:1021–1027.
46 Griffiths PD, Panjwani DD, Stirk PR, et al: Rapid diagnosis of cytomegalovirus infection in immunocompromised patients by detection of early antigen fluorescent foci. Lancet 1984;ii: 1242–1245.
47 Collaborative DHPE Treatment Study Group: Treatment of serious cytomegalovirus infections with 9-(1,3 dihydroxy-2 proproxymethyl) guanine in patients with AIDS and other immunodeficiencies. N Engl J Med 1986;314:801–805.
48 Higgins RM, Bloom SL, Hopkin JM, et al: The risks and benefits of low dose cotrimoxazole prophylaxis for *Pneumocystis pneumonia* in renal transplantation. Transplantation 1989; 47:558–560.
49 Burke CM, Theodore J, Dawkins KD, et al: Post-transplant obliterative bronchiolitis and other late lung sequelae in human heart-lung transplantation. Chest 1984;84:824–829.
50 Burke CM, Theodore J, Baldwin JC, et al: Twenty-eight cases of human heart-lung transplantation. Lancet 1986;i:517–519.
51 Scott JP, Higenbottam TW, Clelland C, et al: The natural history of obliterative bronchiolitis and occlusive vascular disease of patients following heart-lung transplantation. Transplant Proc 1989;21:2592–2593.

Dr. T.W. Higenbottam
Department of Respiratory Physiology
Papworth Hospital
Cambridge CB3 8RE (UK)

Respiration 1991;58(suppl 1):30–33

0025–7931/91/0587–0030 $ 2.75/0

Hyperreactivity and Bronchial Obstruction

S. Bianco, M. Robuschi, P. Sestini

Institutes of Respiratory Diseases of Milano and Siena, Italy

Key Words. Asthma · Chronic obstructive pulmonary disease · Bronchospasm · Hyperreactivity, bronchial · Bronchodilator therapy

Abstract. The main obstructive components in bronchial asthma and chronic obstructive pulmonary disease (COPD) are discussed. It is underscored that bronchospasm plays a significant role also in COPD, and that it merits specific treatment (β_2-stimulants, antimuscarinics, theophylline) even when, in some cases, obstruction appears to be 'irreversible'. The majority of COPD patients react positively, although to a lower degree than asthmatics, not only to chemical agents (histamine, methacholine), but also to 'osmotic' stimuli, such as ultrasonically nebulized distilled water. Geometric factors seem to be in part responsible for the anomalous response. Considering the potent antireactive activity of bronchodilators (β_2-stimulants in particular), this finding is a further indication for a regular bronchodilator treatment in COPD. Whether such a therapy serves also to improve the prognosis of COPD in the long run has not yet been established.

Airflow limitation is commonly observed in bronchial asthma and in the chronic bronchitis-pulmonary emphysema complex or chronic obstructive pulmonary disease (COPD), in which the relative contribution of the two diseases to airflow limitation is practically impossible to establish [1–4]. The main obstructive components in bronchial asthma are bronchospasm, airway wall inflammation, most commonly with eosinophilic infiltration, mucosal edema, and increased secretion. Typically, this form of obstruction is highly reversible either spontaneously or as a result of treatment with bronchospasmolytic drugs, such as β_2-agonists, antimuscarinics, theophyllines, and/or with antiinflammatory agents, such as chromone derivatives and corticosteroids.

In COPD, the obstruction is mainly due to a neutrophilic inflammation of the peripheral airways, destruction of lung parenchyma and mucus hypersecretion [4]. Since bronchial obstruction in these patients fails to respond promptly to bronchospasmolytic agents, bronchospasm is not generally considered to be an important component of bronchial obstruction, which has been misleadingly qualified as 'irreversible'. Consequently, patients with COPD only rarely receive a bronchodilator treatment on a regular basis, despite the fact that a significant 'reversible' component of bronchial obstruction can be demonstrated sooner or later with repeated bronchodilator challenges also in those subjects who first appeared to be unresponsive [5, 6].

Recently, a multicenter, double-blind controlled trial has been performed [7], in which two well-matched groups of relatively stable patients with bronchitis-emphysema were randomly assigned to receive for a period of 5 months (November 1987–April 1988) 2 puffs three times a day of either a combination of fenoterol and ipratropium bromide, 200 and 40 μg/puff, respectively, or a placebo consisting of propellent alone in identical pressurized canisters. At the beginning of the study and at monthly intervals, the patients were subjected to a clinical examination and to respiratory function tests including measurements of PEFR, FEV_1, and MEF25–75. All subjects were equipped with a diary card in which cough, sputum production, and dyspnea were scored daily on a 4-point arbitrary scale. Each patient also received a canister containing fenoterol 200 μg/puff to be used in addition to the experimental treatment in case of dyspnea, recording the number of puffs in the diary card. Corticosteroids, antibiotics, and theophylline were permitted only when strictly necessary during exacerbation phases, and their use was also recorded. In addition, PEFR was recorded every day at 7 a.m. and 7 p.m., immediately before the morning and evening treatments.

At the end of the study, 137 and 139 subjects from the placebo and active-treatment groups, respectively, were found to be suitable for analysis. The results have clearly shown that the bronchodilator treatment induced a consistent increase in all ventilatory parameters in comparison to placebo. Correspondingly, an improvement in the clinical condition, less fenoterol consumption and, in spite of this, less difficulty in breathing were found. It has to be noted that a significant improvement in ventilatory function was observed also in those patients who had shown a low degree of reversibility of the bronchial obstruction (less than 7% of baseline FEV_1) in the preliminary bronchodilator challenge. This stresses the need of bronchodilator treatment even in patients with apparently 'irreversible' airway obstruction.

Bronchial hyperresponsiveness, i.e. the tendency to bronchoconstriction in response to low-intensity nonspecific stimuli, such as cold air, nonisotonic aqueous aerosols, histamine, and methacholine, is a cardinal feature of asthma and relates more closely to the severity of the disease and the need of antiasthmatic treatment than does lung function at rest [8–10]. Results of methacholine and histamine tests are closely correlated, whereas the correlation can be less significant when the responses to chemical and physical stimuli are compared.

Although bronchial hyperresponsiveness is characteristic of asthma, it can also be found in a consistent number of smokers with airflow limitation [11–15]. These subjects are usually less reactive than asthmatics, and the dose-response curve to histamine and methacholine often presents a plateau which is not seen in asthmatics. Other characteristics of bronchial reactivity which are different in the two groups, according to Yan et al. [15], are: (a) Equimolar doses of methacholine and histamine have the same bronchoconstrictor effect in asthmatics, whereas bronchitic smokers are significantly more reactive to histamine than to methacholine. (b) α-Adrenergic stimulation with methoxamine induces bronchoconstriction in asthmatics but almost no response in bronchitics. (c) Patients with COPD tend to be less sensitive to physical stimuli, such as hyperventilation, and do not show any correlation between the responses to cold air and methacholine. (d) A significant inverse correlation is observed between airway caliber and hyperresponsiveness in COPD but not in asthma. According to Ramsdale et al. [12], airway obstruction could account for about 75% of the response to methacholine in bronchitics, but only for 30% in asthmatics.

To further characterize bronchial hyperresponsiveness in smokers with and without airflow limitation, we have devised a study in which the bronchial responses to methacholine and ultrasonically nebulized distilled water (UNW) are compared in smokers with airflow limitation (group SO; FEV_1 >0.8 liters and <80% of predicted), and in control smokers (CS) and nonsmokers (NS; FEV_1 >80% of predicted). So far, we have tested 12 NS, 11 CS, and 6 SO. After a preliminary screening visit, the subjects were challenged with increasing doubling concentrations of methacholine, starting with 0.03 mg/ml in the SO and 0.5 mg/ml in the other groups, up to a highest concentration of 128 mg/ml or until an FEV_1 fall of 20% of baseline was observed. At the same hour of a different and usually not consecutive day, the subjects were then challenged with UNW, starting with 1 ml delivered at the mouth in the SO, and 8 ml in the other groups, up to a cumulated dose of 64 ml. In addition, a second methacholine test was performed 2 h after the end of the UNW challenge, when respiratory parameters had returned to baseline values. The various PC or PD were determined by linear interpolation of the log cumulative dose-response curve. The results of the methacholine challenge showed that most patients in the SO group had marked bronchial hyperresponsiveness. The nonobstructed smokers (CS group) also had a response to methacholine significantly higher than that of the nonsmokers, but to a lower degree than the SO. By contrast, none of the subjects in the NS or CS groups responded to UNW, while about 70% of the SO group presented a 20% decrease in FEV_1 and/or a 100% increase in sR_{aw} upon UNW testing. Furthermore, a significant increase in methacholine reactivity after UNW testing was observed in the SO and CS groups. These results indicate that: (a) patients with COPD might have bronchial hyperresponsiveness even in the absence of a so-called 'reversible component of the obstruction'; (b) the increase in bronchial reactivity to methacholine following UNW challenge is not specific for bronchial asthma but is also observed in COPD and in normal smokers, and (c) the response to UNW appears more specific for COPD than methacholine reactivity, suggesting that sensitivity to physical stimuli might participate in the pathogenesis of the disease. The main practical implication of these results, however, is that bronchodilators could be useful in the treatment of patients with COPD even in the presence of a negative bronchodilator challenge, since they effectively prevent the bronchial hyperresponsiveness which is present in these subjects.

Our results also confirm those of previous cross-sectional studies indicating a significant correlation between airway hyperresponsiveness and the degree of airway obstruction. It has been established from these studies that bronchial hyperreactivity and low baseline FEV_1 are closely related to the accelerated annual decline in FEV_1 observed in patients with COPD. It is not known, however, whether bronchial hyperreactivity plays a primary causative role in this phenomenon, or whether it is secondary to the development of bronchial obstruction. If this is the case, then geometric factors, inflammation, and an increased deposition of bronchoconstrictor aerosols in the central airways could be the operative factors causing bronchial hyperreactivity in these subjects.

Although longitudinal studies are needed to establish whether bronchial hyperreactivity is primary or secondary to bronchial obstruction, nevertheless it most probably represents a risk factor in the pathogenesis of progressive bronchial obstruction. Another risk factor is bronchial and alveolar inflammation. Therefore, it seems that treatments aimed at controlling bronchial reactivity with bronchospasmolitic-antireactive agents and inflammation with inhaled corticosteroids are justified in these patients. We have shown that a 5-month treatment with fenoterol and ipratropium bromide improves both ventilatory function and quality of life. Further studies are needed to establish whether the prognosis of the disease is also improved. Retrospective uncontrolled studies by Postma et al. [16, 17] suggest that the long-term use of oral prednisolone at daily doses >7.5 mg may slow the progression of COPD. Some controlled long-term studies have now been undertaken to determine whether an intervention program with inhaled steroids in combination with β_2-agonists or β_2-agonists and ipratropium is superior to treatment with bronchospasmolytic agents alone, in terms of the annual rate of decline of airway caliber, reversibility of bronchial obstruction, airway hyperreactivity, symptoms, absence from work, days of hospitalization, and quality of life.

References

1 Ciba Guest Symposium: Terminology, definition, and classification of chronic pulmonary emphysema and related conditions. Thorax 1959;14:286–299.
2 Meneely GR, Rensetti AD Jr, Steele JD, Wyatt JP, Harris HW: American Thoracic Society: Chronic bronchitis, asthma, and pulmonary emphysema. Am Rev Respir Dis 1962;85:762–768.
3 Fletcher CM, Pride NB: Definitions of emphysema, chronic bronchitis, asthma, and airflow obstruction: 25 years from the Ciba Symposium. Thorax 1984;39:81–85.
4 Borrows B, Fletcher CM, Heard BE, Jones NL, Wootliff JS: The emphysematous and bronchial types of chronic airways obstruction. Lancet 1966;ii:830–835.
5 Anthonisen NR, Wright EC, Hodgkin JE, IPPB Trial Group: Prognosis in chronic obstructive pulmonary disease. Am Rev Respir Dis 1986;13:14–20.
6 Gross NJ: COPD: A disease of reversible airflow limitation. Am Rev Respir Dis 1986;133:725–726.
7 Bianco S, Olivieri D, Marenco G: Multicenter Italian study of fenoterol and ipratropium bromide (FIMS) for long-term treatment of chronic obstructive pulmonary diseases (COPD). A double-blind, placebo-controlled trial; in Olivieri D, Bianco S (eds): Airway Obstruction and Inflammation. Prog Respir Res. Basel, Karger, 1990, vol 24, pp 243–255.
8 Makino S: Clinical significance of bronchial sensitivity to acetylcholine and histamine in bronchial asthma. J Allergy 1966;38:127–142.
9 Hargreave FE, Ryan G, Thompson NC, et al: Bronchial responsiveness to histamine and methacholine in asthma: Measurements and clinical significance. J Allergy Clin Immunol 1981;68:347–355.
10 Josephs LK, Gregg I, Mullee MA, Holgate ST: Non-specific bronchial reactivity and its relationship to the clinical expression of asthma. A longitudinal study. Am Rev Respir Dis 1989;140:350–357.
11 Ramsdell JW, Nachtwey FJ, Moser KM: Bronchial hyperreactivity in chronic obstructive bronchitis. Am Rev Respir Dis 1982;126:829–832.
12 Ramsdale EH, Morris MM, Roberts RS, Hargreave FE: Bronchial responsiveness to methacholine in chronic bronchitis: Relationship to airflow obstruction and cold air responsiveness. Thorax 1984;39:912–918.
13 Bahous J, Cartier A, Pineau L, et al: Pulmonary function tests and airway responsiveness to methacholine in chronic bronchiectasis of the adult. Bull Eur Physiopathol Respir 1984; 20:375–380.

14 Pride NB, Taylor RG, Lim H, et al: Bronchial hyperresponsiveness as a risk factor for progressive airflow obstruction in smokers. Bull Eur Physiopathol Respir 1987;23:369–375.
15 Yan K, Salome CM, Woolcock AJ: Prevalence and nature of bronchial hyperresponsiveness in subjects with chronic obstructive pulmonary disease. Am Rev Respir Dis 1985;132:25–29.
16 Postma DS, Steenhuis EJ, Van Der Veele LTH, Sluiter HJ: Severe chronic airflow obstruction: Can corticosteroids slow down progression? Eur J Respir Dis 1985;67:56–64.
17 Postma DS, Peters I, Steenhuis EJ, Sluiter HI: Moderately severe airway obstruction: Can corticosteroids slow down obstruction? Eur Respir J 1988;1:22–26.

S. Bianco
Via Cottolengo 42
I-20143 Milano (Italy)

Respiration 1991;58(suppl 1):34–36

0025–7931/91/0587–0034 $ 2.75/0

Management of Bronchial Asthma

Heinrich Matthys

Division of Pneumology, Department of Internal Medicine, University Hospital, Freiburg, FRG

Key Words. Asthma therapy · Bronchial obstruction · Airway hyperreactivity · Inflammation, eosinophilic · Inhalation · Glucocorticoid therapy · Mucociliary clearance · Antiasthmatic drug efficacy

Abstract. The goals of the therapy of bronchial asthma are: (1) freedom from symptoms (within days); (2) normal spirometry (within weeks); (3) reduced or absent hyperreactivity and eosinophilia (within months), and (4) no airway inflammation = normal mucociliary clearance rate ('cured asthma'). Nobody knows how to cure asthma, but we know that we can reach at least stages 1 and 2 with consequent pharmacotherapy, and often also stages 3 and 4 by avoiding asthma-triggering agents and using long-term topical glucocorticoid therapy by inhalation.

Bronchial obstruction, its reversibility, airway hyperreactivity, and eosinophilic inflammation are key variables of asthma. They define different disease states of asthma (table 1) which need different diagnostic and therapeutic measures according to the intensity (severe, light), duration (seasonal, perennial), and etiology (extrinsic, intrinsic, drug induced) of symptoms.

Emergency Treatment of the Acute Attack

The survival rate of patients with severe asthmatic attacks depends critically on the time which passes between the first-aid call and the arrival of the doctor (table 2). Severe asthma may be best defined by functional criteria like the measurement of peak expiratory flow (PEF) $\leqq 100$ l/min and/or a $PaO_2 \leqq 60$ mm Hg, with a $PaCO_2 > 45$ mm Hg. Blood gases are generally only measured under hospital conditions. The amount of wheezing is not a reliable sign to assess the severity of airway obstruction. If PEF does not improve or remains stable within 1–2 h after the start of the emergency treatment, the patient generally needs hospitalization and eventually mechanical ventilation. Hospitalization is often a failure of doctor-patient relationship, e.g. outpatient management. Drugs for sedation who might reduce respiratory drive and/or respiratory muscle force (e.g. Valium) should only be given when mechanical ventilation facilities are immediately available or necessary.

A bolus of prednisolone 50–100 mg i.v. repeated within 2–4 h is the first measure together with aerosol inhalation of a β_2-agonist and eventually an anticholinergic drug in the same metered-dose canister or mechanical nebulizer (table 3). The optimal dose is reached when the patient gets β_2-induced muscle tremor. In patients who are unable to inhale, only systemic β_2-agonists (administered subcutaneously or intravenously) are indicated, because they are weaker bronchodilators (like theophylline) and induce more side effects than when administered by aerosol routes. Systemic theophylline in the form of an oral solution is equally effective in time and duration as an intravenous bolus injection within 10 min. Oral solutions, suppositories, or enemas are administered generally in young children and old adults who have difficulties to inhale or swallow. An alternative for inhalation therapy in these patients are spacers and/or modern dry-powder inhalers as well as mechanical and ultrasonic nebulizers [1]. If the patients are on slow-release tablets, theophylline serum level measurements are often necessary to avoid overdosing with subsequent cardiac arrhythmia, seizures, nausea, and vomiting due to too high or quick infusions. Additional saline solution is given through the initial intravenous route which is kept open for further drug treatment in all patients with severe asthma attacks.

Table 1. Definitions of different disease stages

Symptom	Asthma classification				
	1	2	3	4	5
Obstruction	yes	no	no	no	no
Reversible	yes	no	no	no	no
Hyperreactive	yes	yes	no	yes	no
Decreased MC	yes	yes	yes	no	no
Increased Eos, IgE	yes	yes	yes	no	no

1 = Symptomatic bronchial asthma; 2 = asymptomatic bronchial asthma; 3 = asthmatic bronchitis without hyperreactivity; 4 = essential (constitutional) hyperreactivity; 5 = 'cured' asthma (only anamnestic); MC = mucociliary clearance; Eos = eosinophils.

Table 2. Treatment criteria

Severe asthma	
Functional criteria	
PEF < 100 liters/min	
PaO_2 < 60 mm Hg	
$PaCO_2$ > 45 mm Hg	
Stable or improving with therapy within 1–2 h (PEF control)	→ Home treatment
Deteriorating or not improving with therapy within 1–2 h (PEF control)	→ Hospitalization
'Dangerous' asthma	
Clinically dyspneic, immobilized patient	
Breathing frequency > 50/min	
Cardiac frequency > 130/min	
Wheezing with silent lung	

Table 3. Emergency treatment of bronchial asthma

Prednisolone, 100–200 mg i.v.
β_2-Agonists and parasympathicolytics
Aerosol (Berodual®, Salbutamol®, Ventilat®)
Bricanyl® s.c.; Bronchospasmin® i.v.
Theophylline, 10–20 mg/kg/day
Initially 6 mg/kg i.v. in 10–20 min
20–40 drops p.o. (200–400 mg)
O_2: sedation (Tavegyl®); reanimation (IPPB)

Table 4. Symptomatic and prophylactic antiasthmatic efficacy of drugs

Drugs used	Administration	Symptomatic		Prophylactic	
		R_{aw}	MC	early	late
β_2-Agonists	inhalation	+++	+++	+++	–
	systemic	+	+++	++	–
Anticholinergics	inhalation	++	('+')	+	–
Theophylline	systemic	+	+++	+	–
Steroids					
Oral	systemic	–	+++	(+)	+++
Topic	inhalation	–	++	(++)	++
DSCG, nedocromil	inhalation	–	(+)	(++)	(+)
	systemic	–	?	(+)	(+)
Secretolytics	systemic	–	('+')	–	–

Symptomatic = Symptomatic drug efficacy; R_{aw} = airway resistance; MC = mucociliary clearance; prophylactic = prophylactic protection of the drug in the allergenic early and/or late-phase response; + = positive; – = no effect; ('') = dose-dependent positive or negative; () = only when administered before challenge; ? = unknown.

Symptomatic Long-Term Treatment

Every acute attack needs successive long-term pharmacotherapy with symptomatic and/or prophylactic antiobstructive activity (table 4). Generally a β_2-agonist and/or an anticholinergic drug are given in a metered-dose inhaler in patients with intrinsic asthma. In patients with allergic asthma, especially in children, we prescribe an aerosol canister containing a β_2-agonist and a prophylactic drug (cromolyn or nedocromil). These combinations with β_2-agonists are used at least four times daily together with a topical steroid (beclomethasone, budesonide, or Flumisolid) generally inhaled in the morning and in the evening at home with a spacer after the β_2-combination but before eating. This administration regimen reduces side effects due to topical steroids (hoarseness of the voice, upper-airway fungal infections, and initial cough).

If aerosol administration is difficult or the asthma is not controlled, especially at night, we add slow-release oral β_2-agonists and/or theophylline. Due to circadian rhythms, we give the higher dose before bedtime and the lower dose in the morning. In children, we try also ketotifen twice daily and control the effect by monitoring the early-morning peak flow during 1 month. In patients with difficulties to sleep or with daily sleepiness under ketotifen, we give the whole dose in the evening, which sometimes helps to reduce theophylline side effects or other causes of sleep disturbances.

If a patient needs oral steroids, we try to reduce the evening dose whenever possible and give the higher dose in the morning. Every patient who needs oral steroids also needs a peak flow meter to monitor his airway obstruction. This allows to titrate the amount of steroids according to objective measurements and not to subjective feelings and fears which are not reliable parameters to find the optimal requirements to avoid long-term side effects due to overdosing.

Modern long-acting β_2-agonists (formoterol, salmeterol) given as an aerosol may help to overcome the early-morning dip or the additional inhalation of β_2-agonists or oral theophylline at night.

Prophylactic Measures

In patients with extrinsic asthma, the avoidance of occupational and natural allergens can often completely reduce the asthmatic symptoms. High altitude and dry desert climate cure symptoms of asthma due to house dust mite and often also pollen from plants not growing there. Sea climate has the same benefit especially on islands with poor vegetation and/or ships far away from the allergenic source. This prophylactic measure can also be a test for the etiology of the asthma, e.g. in house dust mite asthma. If a patient does not improve in a climate with low water vapor pressure, the house dust mite allergen is not the leading cause of his asthma symptoms.

Measures in the Symptom-Free Interval

Immunotherapy generally only helps in patients with seasonal symptoms due to only a few leading allergens. Immunotherapy (hypo- or desensitization) reduces symptoms mainly in young patients for a short period of about 3 years if they received the therapy for the same time during their symptom-free interval. Immunotherapy is especially successful in adolescents and children with moderate or light asthma symptoms. About 50% of them loose their asthma also when treated with antiasthmatic drugs alone which in contrast to immunotherapy have practically no mortality.

Surgical treatment, acupuncture, and other physical measures have a more or less pronounced effect on the frequently observed asthmatic symptoms due to conditioned or so-called Pavlov reflexes. They cannot cure asthma because asthma is a genetically transferred disposition for bronchial hyperreactivity nowadays proven by bone marrow transplantation [2]. This has been assumed since years due to the correlation with other atopic diseases.

Bronchial hyperreactivity is a necessary but not sufficient condition for the diagnosis of asthma. The eosinophilic inflammation of the bronchial tree is quantitatively best assessed by measurements of mucociliary clearance. Mucociliary clearance correlates well with measured unspecific (e.g. carbachol) and allergen-induced hyperreactivities and the severity of airway obstruction [3]. Allergen-induced hyperreactivity with its immediate and late-phase airway obstruction reflects better but not completely the clinical picture of asthma. Weekly allergen provocations in allergen-sensitive asthmatics do not lead to the clinical picture of sustained asthmatic symptoms but they increase the nonspecific bronchial hyperreactivity. An increase in nonspecific hyperreactivity is also observed after long-term β_2-agonist therapy compared to topical steroids [4].

Under oral steroid and β_2-agonist therapy, the unspecific hyperreactivity is less reduced compared to the aerosol administration of these drugs at equipotent doses which control the asthmatic symptoms. Hyperreactivity therefore reflects more the severity of the disease and less the therapeutic efficacy of drug treatment. The golden rule for the appropriate asthma treatment remains the daily peak flow protocol and not more or less elaborated relatively seldom applied lung function and/or hyperreactivity measurements which might be necessary to diagnose but not treat asthma adequately.

References

1 Matthys H: Inhalation delivery of asthma drugs. Lung 1990; 168(suppl):645–652.
2 Agosti IM, Sprenger ID, Lum LG, Witherspoon RP, Fischer LD, Storb DR, Henderson WR: Transfer of allergen-specific IgE-mediated hypersensitivity with allogenic bone marrow transplantation. N Engl J Med 1988;319:1623.
3 Matthys H: Definition and assessment of asthma. Lung 1990; 168(suppl):51–56.
4 Kerrebijn KF: Long-term drug treatment of asthma in children. Lung 1990;168(suppl):142–153.

Heinrich Matthys
Division of Pneumology
Department of Internal Medicine
University Hospital
D-W-7800 Freiburg (FRG)

Respiration 1991;58(suppl 1):37–42

0025–7931/91/0587–0037 $ 2.75/0

History of the Treatment of Chronic Bronchitis

Irwin Ziment

Olive View Medical Center, Sylmar, Calif., USA

Key Words. Bronchodilators · Mucokinetic agents · Mucoregulators · Pungent spices · Iodides

Abstract. Although chronic bronchitis was first named and described in 1808, the disease has been known since earliest time, and numerous drugs have been utilized in its therapy. The basic historic theories of human function have readily been applied to bronchitis; thus in Greek medicine, the disease was appreciated as one of excess phlegm. Early remedies included garlic, pepper, cinnamon, and turpentine, whereas later therapies of choice emphasized coffee, ipecac, and potassium nitrate. Most of the favored bronchodilator drugs of today are derived from the traditional folk remedies, ephedrine, atropine, and theophylline. The most interesting historical drugs, however, are those that have given rise to modern mucokinetic agents such as bromhexine and iodides.

Bronchitis was distinguished from other lung disorders such as asthma, catarrh, winter cough, pneumonia and tuberculosis by Charles Badham [1], who named the disease in a book in 1808. Various medical theories over the years have offered complex explanations for the cough, dyspnea, wheezing and expectoration that are characteristic of bronchitis and related diseases [1–22]. However, treatment rarely appears to be based on these explanations, and regimens throughout history have been empirically derived, and were usually based upon plant drugs, inhalation vapors and physical methods such as venesection, skin stimulation and purging.

Ancient Medical Theories

Chinese traditional medicine is based upon the concept of the cosmic opposites yin and yang which control the universal energy, ch'i, and interact to affect the distribution of the five basic elements (wu hsing), which are wood, fire, water, earth and metal or air. Bronchitis is considered to be a result of deficient yin in the lung, and dogma would dictate that therapy be related to this. It is difficult to discern how this concept was ever applied in traditional practice, although acupuncture therapy (rather than herbal remedies) conforms to these theories.

Indian traditional medicine was systematized into the practices of Ayurveda ('science of life'). The basic theory is related to the three fundamental forces (tridosha): kapha which is cold and moist, pitta which is equated with fire, and vata which is related to wind or air. Bronchitis results from an excess of kapha, and remedies were usually based on plant extracts which allegedly had pitta and vata qualities.

Greek-Roman ideas on disease had some resemblance to Indian concepts and each probably was derived from Mesopotamian practices that arose from magical and religious ceremonies. In Greece, the philosophic teachings of *Alcmaeon* of Croton, *Pythagoras,* and *Empedocles* of Acragas led to the lasting Hippocratic belief that there were four humors and corresponding qualities: phlegm which was equated with cold and moist qualities, blood which was hot and moist, yellow bile which was hot and dry, and black bile which was cold and dry. This theory would suggest that excess phlegm in bronchitis would require a hot, dry remedy such as pepper. However, actual practice had an empirical basis, and thus, an odd collection of plants such as sweetflag, pellitory, mandrake, bryony and so forth were included in *Dioscorides'* recommendations for bronchitis.

In each major medical system, it was believed that the underlying energy of the universe entered the body as air. The vital component of air was called ch'i by the Chinese, ruach by the Hebrews, prana by the Indians, and pneuma by the Greeks. In Greek-Roman pneumatist thinking, the pneuma interacted with food (chyle) and blood, thus forming natural spirit in the liver, vital spirit in the heart and animal spirit in the brain. *Hippocrates* thought that excess phlegm would flow (as rheum) from the brain and be discharged as pituita or catarrh. It was not until *van Helmont* in the 17th century discredited these ideas that the stage was set for bronchitis to be seen as a disease originating in the lower respiratory tract.

Ancient Therapies

In general, most of the accepted ancient treatments had little relationship to the theories of disease. The *Mesopotamians* used numerous drugs, many of which were strong smelling, to drive the 'evil' out of the lungs. Some were used as nauseants and emetics, others as inhalants, and others with no clear rationale. The *Akkadians* may have been the first to use belladonna, although the related mandrake was more favored as it was thought to have magical properties.

Subsequently, the *Egyptians,* as an outgrowth of their strong interests in incenses, perfumes, cosmetics and embalming, introduced an increased range of inhalational drugs. However, the Ebers Papyrus (1600 BC) gave the following placebo prescription for asthma: fig, grape, sycamore fruit, frankincense, cumin, juniper, goosegrease, wine and beer. Subsequently, the *Hebrews* showed disenchantment with all drug therapy, but used a number of spices and herbs in their ceremonial incenses. The famous biblical incense drugs, such as myrrh, galbanum, cinnamon, calamus and frankincense, were to enter popular medicine in later years as expectorants. But the only agent recommended as an expectorant in biblical commentaries was the onion.

Greek-Roman Therapies

The prevailing belief that illness resulted from abnormal humors encouraged the Greeks to employ bleeding and purging and to give emetics in many diseases. Bleeding may have helped the bronchitis patient who had pulmonary edema or polycythemia, while emetics could certainly be of value in inducing mucokinesis.

Hippocrates (460–370 BC) wisely avoided most drugs, but he had little to say about asthma and bronchitis. He used honey in water (hydromel) or in vinegar (oxymel) for many pulmonary disorders, but he wrote that water does not promote expectoration. Inhalation therapy was resorted to for 'draining the lungs', using warmed mixtures of fruit juice, salt, grease, flower juice and vinegar. Hyssop was used, and remained popular as an expectorant subsequently, although it does not appear to be effective.

Dioscorides in the 1st century AD wrote *De Materia Medica,* and described over 600 plants; many mucokinetic agents still in use date back to his authority, e.g. coltsfoot *(Tussilago farfara),* comfrey, elecampane, horehound, marshmallow, mullein, pepper, radish and squill.

Pliny the Elder in the 1st century AD collected information from wide-ranging sources and commented on numerous drugs. Of interest was the report of Majno [6] that Pliny wrote about the plant ephedron, which was probably a European Ephedra, that may have yielded ephedrine. This was recommended by Pliny for cough, asthma, colic and to arrest nasal bleeding. However, the drug did not receive subsequent attention in Europe until the 1920s.

Galen (131–201 AD) had little to add to previous ideas, although he may have produced asthma experimentally. He prescribed attenuant and detergent medicines to loosen mucus, but confused both dogma and fact by suggesting that both hot and cold material might thicken the phlegm.

Aretaeus the Cappadocian (who gave one of the first good descriptions), *Aetius, Actuarius, Aurelianus* and *Aegineta* were some of the physicians who wrote about asthma and bronchitis. They recommended a mixture of diet, drugs, clysters, poultices, venesection, cupping, scarification, inhalations, formentations, sponging, baths, massaging, exercise, travel, change in climate and so on – and thus offered a foundation of holistic and ridiculous practices that was to dominate in therapeutics for well over 1,000 years.

Therapy in the Middle Ages

The most famous medieval book on asthma was *Maimonides'* treatise written in 1190. In spite of offering general sensible holistic advice, the book restates Galenic Greek-Roman concepts and uses a mixture of ancient and new placebo remedies. Furthermore, Maimonides gave some very poor and contradictory suggestions. Thus, at one point he condemns warm spices, then later recommends the use of green pepper, coriander, ginger, cloves, onions and mustard. He recognized the value of emetic therapy, but many of his botanic remedies were probably placebos, e.g. liquirita, althaea, fleabane, fennel, wheat bran and almond oil. It is unclear why he condemned other foods and plants, such as lettuce, pumpkin, cauliflower, turnip, peach, apricot, cucumber and date. He also disdained onion and garlic, but his other writings on poisoning offer the rationale that such highly flavored foods could disguise a hidden poison prepared by a malignant schemer. Maimonides gained lasting fame by recommending chicken soup, but his recipe is of dubious merit: he used fat old hens, and added such components as rice, beans and spikenard in addition to spice flavor agents such as coriander, ginger, cloves, mint, lemon juice and vinegar.

Paracelsus, Cardano and *van Helmont* gradually helped bring more rationalism, but still mixed with medieval fancies, into therapeutics during the Renaissance. Thus, Cardano may have recognized that asthma could be caused by feathers, although his rigorous regimen of strict diet, cold bathing and exercise in cold rainy weather may have helped induce bronchitis. Van Helmont, an asthmatic himself, recognized to some extent the concept of hypersensitivity and believed that chemical and physical injury to the lungs caused disease, which could then be self-perpetuating. His comparison of asthma to epilepsy was equally insightful, although his treatment remained rooted in traditionalism as modified by Paracelsus.

Pre-Modern Therapeutics

Thomas Willis [20], in the 17th century, provided one of the first relatively scientific accounts of asthma, and recognized that wheezing and dyspnea were caused by spasm of the bronchial muscles. However, most of his therapeutic suggestions were based on traditional nonsense. Thus, he recommended, reasonably, a prescription of horehound, garlic, saffron and castoreum. Less acceptable is his inclusion in other prescriptions of numerous useless plant derivatives, and more ridiculous things such as preparations from millipedes, earthworms and snails. Of interest is his use of expensive spices from the Orient such as long pepper, cubebs, cloves and mace. Of greatest interest is his neo-Maimonidean recommendation that herbal mixtures should be sewn up in an old cock and boiled to make a soup.

John Floyer [4], an asthmatic himself, in the late 17th century wrote more extensively on asthma, and differentiated between several acute and chronic diseases, and the various etiologic factors such as emotion and chemical irritation. However, his prescriptions ranged from the acceptable to the ludicrous. Many of his dietary and drug recommendations were similar to those of Maimonides and Willis, but he was a strong advocate of purging and cold bathing. An interesting treatment was friction massage of the legs and thighs. Also of interest, he advocated avoiding a mucilaginous diet, since he believed phlegm was thickened by fish, legumes and milk.

William Withering in 1786 wrote an essay on *The Spasmodic Asthma* [8], in which he demonstrated familiarity with standard holistic advice, but he avoided harmful measures such as venesection. He advised long sea or land journeys, exercise, cold fresh air and baths, and sleeping on a mattress without feathers in a large room without curtains while keeping the legs warm and the head high. However, his drug therapy was less enlightened, consisting of agents such as tar, assafetida and oil of amber, and also opium to relieve fits. He was perhaps the earliest major advocate of very strong coffee.

Charles Badham [1] in 1808 wrote his book in which he named the entity of bronchitis. However, his therapies were not innovative: venesection, blistering of the chest, purgatives, sudorifics and expectorants, particularly antimonials and ipecacuanha. Being an Englishman, he recognized that 'nothing does so much good as a change of air'.

Henry Salter [15] who was to die of asthma at the age of 44, in 1859 wrote an important article on asthma, in which he examined all current theories, including the possibility that the disorder in many cases was the 'dyspnea of bronchitis'. In his book on asthma in 1860, he enthusiastically advocated stramonium, nitre, lobelia and coffee. He believed asthma was worse in sleep, and thus reasoned that very strong, black coffee was indicated, whereas the relatively popular use of opium was inappropriate. However, he also recommended tobacco, which could be dosed to produce sedative or depressant effects; if pushed ad nauseam, he claimed it gave more relief in hay-asthma than any other remedy. Surprisingly, Salter was convinced that city air – particularly the smokiest – was good for some asthmatics, but he did not allude to the danger of bronchitis. He did not advocate seaside air, nor did he think potassium iodide was useful.

The Modern Era

Current drugs for bronchitis include the adrenergic bronchodilators, theophylline, corticosteroids, anticholinergics, expectorants, oxygen and antibiotics. The history of these (except for oxygen and antibiotics) will be briefly presented.

Adrenergics

The Chinese have used Ma huang from *Ephedra sinensis* for coughs, fevers and edema for thousands of years, but it was not clearly used to treat asthma until this century. In the 1920s, Cheng and Schmidt demonstrated that the plant product contained ephedrine which they proved to be a bronchodilator.

Adrenaline was isolated from the adrenal gland following the original studies of Oliver in 1893 in Harrogate; in 1897 this extract was recognized to be a 'hormone'. It was called epinephrine by Abel of Johns Hopkins in 1897, and was subsequently renamed adrenaline by Takamine who found a method of purifying it. Solis-Cohen [18] of Philadelphia had recommended oral adrenal substance (5 grains) for treating bronchospasm in 1900. Adrenaline became more popular when the pure solution was given by aerosol in 1929 at Guy's Hospital. The next adrenergic to be introduced for asthma, isoproterenol, did not appear until 1951.

Theophylline

Although coffee had been repeatedly described (by Withering, Laennec, Trousseau, Floyer, Salter and Trendelenberg among others) as of benefit in asthma since the 18th century, tea has not been described as a valuable remedy. However, in 1888 Kossel isolated from tea, and named, theophylline (which means 'tealeaf'); in 1908, theophylline ethylenediamine (aminophylline) was introduced. In 1921, theophylline was shown to be a bronchodilator, and its value as a treatment for asthma when given rectally was shown soon after. In 1927, aminophylline was first given intravenously for asthma. It is of interest that today the value of theophylline is being questioned in both asthma and bronchitis, and it may in fact be more valuable in the latter disease.

Glucocorticoids

In 1948, a series of serendipitous events led to the introduction of cortisone by Hench at the Mayo Clinic for the treatment of rheumatoid arthritis. The reasoning that suggested the use of an adrenal hormone was based on the observation that pregnancy results in improvement of arthritis. However, this does not occur with asthma, and thus if Hench had been a pulmonologist, he would not have tried cortisone therapy. Indeed, oral extracts of adrenal cortex had been given by previous investigators without much observable benefit in asthma. Nevertheless, steroid preparations were eventually tried in numerous diseases, including asthma; nowadays, they are used far more for asthma than for arthritis, where nonsteroidal drugs are preferred. Eventually, the same change in therapy may occur with asthma; in bronchitis, this is even more likely, since steroids are of variable and dubious value in this disorder.

Anticholinergics

It is probable that various solanaceous plants were used in asthma and bronchitis in early Mesopotamian medicine, but their true value seems to have only gradually been recognized in India. There, the plant called dhatura in Sanskrit was utilized in burning powders for centuries before the English brought *Datura stramonium* cigarettes to England for the treatment of asthma. Atropine was isolated from *Atropa belladonna* roots by Mein in 1833, and gradually this became an accepted drug for the treatment of asthma. In 1859, Courty [15] claimed to have relieved an asthmatic attack by injecting the vagus nerve with atropine. With the introduction of ipratropium in 1968, anticholinergic therapy was gradually recognized to be of greater value in bronchitis and emphysema than in asthma. The second major component of Atropa is hyoscine, also known as scopolamine, since it was obtained from *Scopola carniolica,* which is named in honor of Scopoli, the 18th-century botanist of the University of Pavia.

Mucokinetics

The vast majority of agents that have been used for respiratory disorders, including asthma and bronchitis, are without significant effects in their customary doses. However, it is probable that many of them, especially in larger doses, can stimulate increased mucokinesis and enhance expectoration by initiating the gastropulmonary vagal emetic-mucokinetic reflex. A few of the well-known agents will be discussed.

Volatile Inhalants. These have been used in all ancient societies, and numerous formulations have been given by various techniques. Some of the most favored include pine products, benzoin, storax, thymol, camphor, eucalyptus, lemon grass, geranium, and spices such as cinnamon and cloves. The balsams - such as benzoin, storax, Tolu balsam and Peruvian balsam - have also been given in oral medications. They continue to be used in many proprietary preparations, although proof of their value has not been given.

Iodide. Seaweed has had a long popularity, and was greatly favored by Laennec, who himself had both asthma and tuberculosis. Iodine was isolated in 1812, and various synthetic products have been introduced since. The most popular mucokinetic is potassium iodide, which may have multiple modes of action. Currently, organic iodides are preferred.

Beechwood Tar. Various woods, including beechwood, contain phenolic products such as creosote and guaiacol. These agents were widely used in the 19th century as oral disinfectants, and they were thought to be particularly useful for pulmonary infections. Indeed, Thiokol (potassium guiacol-sulfonate) was the first marketing success of Hoffmann-La Roche. Currently, guaifenesin is the most popular over-the-counter mucokinetic in the USA, although conventional doses are subtherapeutic in most cases.

Pine Products. The resins from pine and larch trees have been valued medicaments for thousands of years. Terebinthus from the turpentine tree was a major trading product, and was used by the Greeks in the treatment of dyspnea. The popular old product that is still used today is terpin hydrate, although this is generally thought to be ineffective. Of greater current interest, sobrerol is a terpenic compound that is synthesized from alpha-pinene, and it is a favored mucokinetic in Europe.

Ipecacuanha. The Portuguese brought back this Brazilian plant to Europe in the 16th century, and it became a popular panacea. It is still valued as an emetic, and in subemetic doses it is useful as a mucokinetic. The popular Indian plant, Tylophora, has similar properties.

Vasaka. This traditional remedy is obtained from the malabar nut of India *(Adhatoda vasika)* and was used for the treatment of asthma and tuberculosis. Modern derivatives include bromhexine, a mucoregulator, and ambroxol, a mucokinetic agent that stimulates surfactant production.

Garlic. This pungent herb has long been used in medicine as an anti-infective and as a mucokinetic. It contains S-allyl-*L*-cysteine sulfoxide (alliin) which on reduction is converted to S-allyl-*L*-cysteine (desoxyalliin). This is similar in chemical composition to S-carboxymethylcysteine, the popular mucoregulator, which is found in nature in radish seedlings. It is probable that the sulfur volatiles of alliaceous plants such as garlic serve both as expectorants and mucoregulators.

Chicken Derivatives. The modern equivalent to the chicken soup of Maimonides and Willis is acetylcysteine, since the cysteine component is derived from chicken feathers and skin. Although the product has chemical resemblance to desoxyalliin in garlic, the latter has a blocked sulfur group and is not a mucolytic. In contrast, acetylcysteine is the most potent mucolytic marketed, and it also offers the additional advantages of being an expectorant, a mucoregulator and an antioxidant.

Selected and Commented Bibliography

1 Badham C: Observations on the inflammatory affections of the mucous membrane of the bronchiae. London, J. Callow, 1808 (in this book, Badham is the first to use the term 'bronchitis').

2 Capel LH: A history of the pulmonary catarrhs and airway obstruction. Br J Dis Chest 1966;60:113.

3 Cosman MP: A feast for Aesculapius. Historical diets for asthma and sexual pleasure. Ann Rev Nutr 1983;3:1.

4 Floyer J: Medicina Geromica. London, J. Isted, 1724 (see chapt 14: 'The Regimen in the Asthma').

5 Gravenstein JS, Kalhan S, Balamoutsos NG: Of breaths and spirits. JAMA 1981;246:1091.

6 Majno G: The Healing Hand. Cambridge, Harvard University Press, 1975 (see pp 349-353 for Majno's discovery of Pliny's information on ephedron).

7 Major RH: A note on the history of asthma; in Underwood EA (ed): Science, Medicine and History. New York, Arno Press, 1975, pp 518-529.

8 Mann RD: Modern Drug Use. Lancaster, MTP Press Limited, 1984 (pp 355-362 provide new information on Withering's 'The Spasmodic Asthma').

9 Marketos SG, Eftychiades A: Bronchial asthma according to Byzantine medicine. J Asthma 1986;23:149.

10 Rosenblatt MB: History of bronchial asthma; in Weiss EB, Segal MS (eds): Bronchial Asthma. Mechanics and Therapeutics. Boston, Little, Brown, 1976, chapt 1.

11 Rosner F: Moses Maimonides' Treatise on Asthma. J Asthma 1984;21:119.

12 Sakula A: John Floyer's 'A Treatise of the Asthma'. Thorax 1984;39:248.

13 Sakula A: Henry Hyde Salter: A biographical sketch. Thorax 1985;40:887.
14 Sakula A: A history of asthma. J R Coll Phys Lond 1985;22:36.
15 Salter HH: An enquiry into the tenability of the various theories of asthma. Edin Med J 1859;5:219 (see also Courty MA in same journal, p 668, on injecting the vagus nerve with atropine to relieve asthma).
16 Schultze-Werminghaus G, Meier-Sydow J: The clinical and pharmacological history of theophylline. Clin Allergy 1982;12: 211.
17 Sneader W: Drug Discovery: The Evolution of Modern Medicine. Chichester, Wiley, 1985 (an extraordinary detailed account).
18 Solis-Cohen S: The use of adrenal substance in the treatment of asthma. JAMA 1900;34:1164.
19 Stolkind E: History of bronchial asthma. Janus 1933;37:300.
20 Willis T: Of the asthma; in: The London Practice of Physick, 1692.
21 Ziment I: Five thousand years of attacking asthma: An overview. Respir Care 1986;31:117.
22 Ziment I: Historic overview of mucoactive drugs; in Braga PC, Allegra L (eds): Drugs in Bronchial Mucology. New York, Raven Press, 1989, chapt 1 (see also chapt 5.7, 7 and 8).

Irwin Ziment, MD
Olive View Medical Center
14445 Olive View Drive
Sylmar, CA 91342-1495 (USA)

Respiration 1991;58(suppl 1):43–46

0025–7931/91/0587–0043 $ 2.75/0

Chronic Bronchitis in the 1990s: Up-To-Date Treatment

S.W. Clarke

Royal Free Hospital, London, UK

Key Words. Chronic bronchitis · Smoking · Drug treatment · Oxygen · Pulmonary rehabilitation

Abstract. Prevention is the key to eradicating chronic bronchitis. Smoking is the prime factor involved. Quitting smoking is difficult even with modern aids such as counselling, filters, substitutes, hypnosis and acupuncture, and the success rate is only 20%. Passive smoking is also injurious. The role of atmospheric pollution is less well quantified. Other risk factors include lower social class, occupation, area of residence, housing, temperature, and childood respiratory illness. Influenza vaccination gives 60–70% immunity. With exacerbations of chronic bronchitis, β-lactamase-producing bacteria are important, though the overall need for antibiotics is uncertain judging by placebo-controlled studies. Inhaled β_2-agonist bronchodilators may improve airflow obstruction, as may anticholinergic drugs (e.g. ipratropium), the two being additive. Oral theophyllines have a narrow therapeutic window, serious side-effects and only two thirds of the effect of β_2-agonists. A corticosteroid trial for 2 weeks may relieve refractory airway obstruction in 17–23% of chronic bronchitics, to be followed by inhaled steroids. Mucolytic drugs remain controversial and are difficult to monitor successfully. Oxygen therapy may be indicated for hypoxic chronic bronchitis, including long-term usage in cor pulmonale. Pulmonary rehabilitation by exercise training has recently been appreciated, and may be used in combination with the above treatment modalities.

The management of chronic bronchitis, which is perhaps a more suitable title, has in fact changed little over the past decade or more. It may be looked at from several aspects: (1) prevention, perhaps the most important aspect, (2) actual treatment with drugs (e.g. bronchodilators) and (3) rehabilitation, the centrepiece of which is the ability to exercise leading to an independent life for the patient.

Prevention of Chronic Bronchitis

Smoking cessation remains the most important step in preventing the progression of chronic bronchitis. Symptoms such as cough and sputum may clear and airway obstruction improve or deteriorate at a slower pace than before [1].

To stop smoking is often not easy for the patient and it always requires a great effort of self-will. There are many ways in which the patient can be helped to stop, the most important being counselling. A variety of other means have been tried, e.g. the use of graduated filters, substitutes such as nicotine chewing gum and sprays, hypnosis, acupuncture or smoking clinics [2]. With all this help and the best will in the world, the relapse rate remains high with a success rate on average of 20% at one year.

The role of atmospheric pollution appears to be substantial in urban areas with high pollution as opposed to rural areas with cleaner air. However, this is less well quantified, and the rural environment is now no longer as clean as it was.

Two other adverse features concerning smoking include the now proven effects of passive smoking, whereby others inhale the smokers' smoke, and there now seems no doubt that this can have deleterious effects on the recipients' lung, a fact which has always seemed likely. The second is that the number of people smoking has fallen progressively over the past years until recently when there has been an increase in the UK, albeit small, but involving young people. This is an ominous return of a bad habit in people who have clearly not responded to the health warnings now given on all cigarette packets, and which appears to be related to lower cost [3]. Other risk factors include social class, occupation, area of residence, housing, temperature, and childhood respiratory illness [4].

Vaccination may be included under the heading of prevention, and this is given principally for influenza, which has a mortality of 1-2/10,000 cases/year. It gives a success rate of 60-70% with a febrile-reaction rate of about 2%, which may be an embarrassment if it occurs. Many doctors give this vaccination routinely in chronic bronchitics.

The value of pneumococcal vaccine, which is also 70% effective, is more controversial in so far as it has not been shown to reduce exacerbations as yet. Nevertheless, since pneumococcal infection in the lung is prevalent in chronic bronchitics, it seems not unreasonable to consider this possibility.

Vaccines against *Haemophilus influenzae* type B and *Pseudomonas aeruginosa* have been formulated, but the former is used for children under the age of 5 years and the latter has not been explored fully [5]. Several oral vaccines of mixed linage are available in Europe, but their efficacy remains unproven.

Long-term chemotherapy has been studied, and although it may reduce exacerbations of chronic bronchitis, nevertheless it does not appear to have any lasting effect and is not in general use.

Treatment of Chronic Bronchitis

Conventionally, exacerbations of chronic bronchitis are treated with an appropriate antibiotic [6]. The causative organisms for exacerbations are often viruses of varying types and are thus not specifically responsive to antibiotics, although subsequent bacterial infection is. The most prevalent bacteria are *Streptococcus pneumoniae, H. influenzae* and a newer one known as *Branhamella catarrhalis.* Both latter organisms may be β-lactamase producers and thus may require treatment with a drug combination such as amoxicillin plus clavulanic acid. Otherwise, tetracycline, ampicillin and trimethoprim are the drugs most commonly used.

The indications for giving antibiotics appear to be perfectly straightforward and include the presence of cough, purulent sputum, fever and dyspnoea. However, when this is looked at more rigorously, it will be noted that many trials to determine the value of antibiotic treatment in acute exacerbations of chronic bronchitis have found no benefit from antibiotic treatment [6]. For example, in a recent study [7] exacerbations were followed in a group of 173 patients with chronic bronchitis over a 3.5-year period, the treatment consisting of antibiotic or placebo administered in a randomised double-blind cross-over fashion.

Three levels of severity of exacerbation were noted, the most severe comprising increasing dyspnoea plus increased sputum volume and purulence, with the other two grades of lesser severity. Amoxicillin and co-trimoxazole were used each in 40%, and doxycycline in the remaining 20%. Of the 362 exacerbations, 182 were treated with antibiotics and 180 with placebo. A successful outcome was judged by resolution of symptoms after 21 days, and this occurred in 55% of the placebo- and 68% of the antibiotic-treated exacerbations. However, the overall failure rate was higher in the placebo (42%) than in the antibiotic group (29%). Placebo appeared to be as good as antibiotics in a less severe category of exacerbation, becoming less so as severity increased, with total failure rates of 53 and 34% in the placebo and antibiotics group, respectively, in the most severe category. Nevertheless, bearing all in mind, this study group considers antibiotics to be justified in such patients with dyspnoea, sputum and purulence, while acknowledging that the underlying cause of the exacerbations is unknown.

Other studies have tried to define the role of infection in an exacerbation, but it is known that up to 80% of patients with chronic bronchitic are colonised with *H. influenzae* or *S. pneumoniae* so that routine sputum culture is virtually valueless [8]. A rising viral antibody titre has been found particularly in male chronic bronchitics who seem susceptible to minor virus infections associated with exacerbations.

Thus the need for antibiotic treatment remains questionable, it seems reasonable to treat the individual case with purulent sputum, but it should be remembered that in 50% of exacerbations the same response and end results will be achieved without antibiotics.

Bronchodilators

β_2-Agonists

Chronic obstructive pulmonary disease is usually poorly reversible, and by definition reversibility is < 15–20% in spirometric indices (FEV_1or PFR). Nevertheless, this response can often be elicited by inhaled aerosol β-agonist bronchodilators, which usually prove more effective than the tablet form. There may be dose-related response [9]; the benefit of this 15–20% increase in flow may be quite marked in the individual patient, and give worthwile reduction of dyspnoea and improvement in exercise tolerance. There does not appear to be tachyphylaxis, and many patients take β-agonists regularly.

Anticholinergic Drugs

The chief member of this group is now ipratropium bromide [10] which is a good bronchodilator equipotent with a β-agonist, though there appear to be patients who are responders and those who are non-responders, the distinction between the two being difficult to pinpoint without a therapeutic trial. The previously feared side-effects are few, and there is no serious reduction in mucociliary clearance [11].

When used in conjunction with β-agonists, the joint bronchodilation is increased, and this combination can be useful over a prolonged period [12].

Theophyllines

This group of drugs has been known for its bronchodilator effects in asthma for many years [13]. Its efficacy in patients with chronic obstructive pulmonary disease is controversial. Short-term improvements have not been found. With long-term treatment, an improvement in the 12 min walking test was equalled by response to a β-agonist. The two drugs together produced a further spirometric response, but were without effects on exercise tolerance. The effect of theophyllines on diaphragmatic contractility is still disputed.

In a recent, dose-related study, theophylline produced no improvement in respiratory function tests, no correlation between dosage and improvement in walking distance and no subjective reduction in the degree of breathlessness assessed by visual-analogue score.

Any improvement with theophylline is probably only two thirds of that achieved with β-stimulants. Theophylline has several drawbacks; its narrow therapeutic margin, its variable pharmacogenetics and its clearance affected by age, smoking, cor pulmonale, respiratory viral infections, impaired liver function, and erythromycin. Toxic effects may be serious and include grand mal seizures with confusion of the patient about the dose prescribed, excessive drug prescription and unrecognised interaction with other drugs.

Most patients fare better with a dose of inhaled bronchodilator that achieves maximum effect both acutely and with maintenance treatment. On occasion, a trial of theophylline may be indicated to improve this effect.

Corticosteroids

Corticosteroids may be expected to relieve airway obstruction if that is partly dependent on bronchoconstriction and inflammatory changes [14]. Several studies have been done using a 2-week course of steroids, and response rates of 17–23% have been achieved. However, the response to steroids cannot be predicted reliably. A response may be predicted if there are features of asthma with an acute increase in FEV_1 after administration of a bronchodilator, spontaneous variability of FEV_1 and blood eosinophilia. Those features of extensive emphysema which include a low gas transfer and collapse of airways on the expiratory flow volume curve indicate that a response is less likely. A decline in $FEV_1 > 80$ ml/year in smokers indicates possible reversibility.

The response to steroids is usually accepted as a 15–20% increase in spirometric indices. Changes in the 12 min walking distance test are variably related to changes in airflow.

Most responses are found to be complete by the 8th day and all by the 11th day, and consequently, a 2-week period is usually given; this can always be extended if thought necessary. The dosage is prednisolone 30–40 mg daily, although there is little evidence on which to base this dosage. In some studies, inhaled steroids have identified most responders, often with some further improvement with prednisolone later.

After a positive trial of steroids, the usual policy is to gradually withdraw prednisolone while introducing inhaled steroids, though in some cases a small maintenance dose may be necessary.

If there has been no effect, then the steroids can be stopped, since pituitary and adrenal function return to normal within 3 days after stopping prednisolone 40 mg daily for 3 weeks. It is possible that steroids may retard disease progression and also damp down airway responsiveness.

Mucolytic drugs remain controversial, insofar as their therapeutic benefit is difficult to prove in clinical studies [15]. This subject is dealt with in detail elsewhere.

Oxygen Therapy

In patients with hypoxaemia either at rest or on exercise, short-term O_2 gives variable effects on exercise tolerance, partly offset by the energy requirements of carrying portable O_2. Furthermore, responders and non-responders can only be distinguished by trial and error [16]. The requirements for long-term O_2 therapy are dealt with elsewhere.

Pulmonary Rehabilitation

Recently, the importance of pulmonary rehabilitation by exercise training has been recognised, and a variety of programmes formulated [17]. Exercise to moderate breathlessness is the key aim. The positive results include improvement in locomotion, physical and psychological independence, and improvement in the quality of life. Simultaneously, full assessment of the patient is carried out, current therapy checked, and smoking discussed.

Conclusion

It is now realised that the well-being and mobility of patients with chronic obstructive bronchitis can be much improved with a combination of the above methods of treatment and management. The new positive approach to these patients is now beginning. Whether long term mortality will be influenced remains to be seen.

References

1 Buist AS, Sexton GJ, Nagy JM, Ross BB: The effect of smoking cessation and modification on lung function. Am Rev Respir Dis 1976;114:115-122.
2 Raw M: The treatment of cigarette dependence; in Israel Y, Glaser FB, Kalant H, et al (eds): Advances in Alcohol Research and Drug Problems, vol 4. New York, Plenum Press, 1978, pp 441-485.
3 Cigarette smoking increases (editorial). Br Med J 1989; 298:12-72.
4 Holland WW: Chronic obstructive lung disease prevention. Br J Dis Chest 1988;82;32-44.
5 Stanley PJ, Ellis CJ: New vaccines. Br J Hosp Med 1989;41: 364-367.
6 Antibiotics for exacerbations of chronic bronchitis? (editorial). Lancet 1987;ii:23-24.
7 Anthonisen NR, Manfreda J, Warren CPW, et al: Antibiotic therapy in exacerbations of chronic obstructive pulmonary disease. Ann Intern Med 1987;106:196-204.
8 Gump DW, Phillips CA, Forsyth BR, et al: Role of infection in chronic bronchitis. Am Rev Respir Dis 1976;113:465-474.
9 Vathenen AS, Britton JR, Ebden P, et al: High-dose inhaled albuterol in severe chronic airflow limitation. Am Rev Respir Dis 1988;138:850-855.
10 Gross NJ: Anticholinergic agents in chronic bronchitis and emphysema. Postgrad Med J 1987;63(suppl 1):29-34.
11 Taylor RG, Pavia D, Agnew JE, et al: Effect of four weeks' high-dose ipratropium bromide treatment on lung mucociliary clearance. Thorax 1986;41:295-300.
12 Bianco S. Olivieri D, Marenco G: Multicenter Italian study of fenoterol and Ipratropium Bromide (FIMS) for long-term treatment of chronic obstructive pulmonauf diseases (COPD); in Olivieri D, Bianco S (eds): Airway Obstruction and Inflammation. Prog Resp Res. Basel, Karger, 1990, p 24, pp 243-255.
13 Slow-release theophyllines and chronic bronchitis (editorial). Br Med J 1984;289:1643-1644.
14 Corticosteroids in chronic bronchitis (editorial). Br Med J 1984; 288:1553-1554.
15 Pavia D: Effects of pharmacologic agents on the clearance of airway secretions. Semin Respir Med 1984;5:345-352.
16 Light RW, Mahutte CK, Stansbury DW, et al: Relationship between improvement in exercise performance with supplemental oxygen and hypoxic ventilatory drive in patients with chronic airflow obstruction. Chest 1989;95;751-756.
17 Cockroft A: Pulmonary rehabilitation. Br J Dis Chest 1988;82; 220-225.

Dr. S.W. Clarke
Royal Free Hospital
Hampstead
London NW3 2QG (UK)

Respiration 1991;58(suppl 1):47–51

0025–7931/91/0587–0047 $ 2.75/0

Mucus Pharmacology

P.C. Braga

Center for Respiratory Pharmacology, School of Medicine, University of Milan, Italy

Key Words. Mucus pharmacology · Muco-active drugs classification · Limiting factors · New schedule

Abstract. Until recently the experimental and clinical possibilities for investigation of the pharmacological effects of drugs acting on airway secretions were limited. Nowadays, new biological, physical and chemical techniques of investigation are applied to 'mucology', providing better characterization of this class of drugs. Experimental and clinical approaches are described.

Primitive societies paid close attention to diseases accompanied by abnormal secretions, and through the centuries, each major civilization has experimented with the plant, mineral and animal products present in its geographic area. In a very exhaustive and quite interesting historic overview of mucoactive drugs, Ziment [1] reported that a huge number of ancient medications have been collected over time; some of those agents, which were already used two or three thousand years ago, stand up to the close examination of modern pharmacology and have been introduced into current respiratory therapy. Some others were mixtures of strange ingredients with no predictable effects, and much of the evidence concerning their clinical value was mainly subjective and based only on 'traditional use' [2].

Until recently, the experimental and clinical possibilities for investigation of the pharmacological effects of a drug acting on airway secretions were quite limited. Nowadays, new biological, physical and chemical techniques of investigation, involving biochemical identification and measurement of the mucus components, and mainly the better determination of rheological parameters and precise evaluation of mucociliary clearance in animals and man are applied to mucology, providing better characterization of this class of drugs. Since the increase in mucus production and changes in physico-chemical properties are defensive reflex responses to noxious biological, chemical and physical stimuli, the primary therapeutic maneuver is to remove the offending cause.

This is obvious, but often not very easy to achieve in clinical practice, so mucostasis is corrected by the use of drugs that fluidize the mucus and improve the clearance of the airways.

Over the years, the discovery of new agents has resulted in new terms being coined to explain their activity on mucus. Year after year, the terminology continues to increase considerably, reflecting the personal background, imagination and individual intention of investigators and clinicians.

As shown in table 1 [3], many terms are used to explain the same properties with only minor semantic differences; so confusion arises, and there is a need to bring some order into this group of drugs, which resulted in various classifications being proposed.

No rigid pharmacological classification of these agents can be offered, as can be for other kinds of drugs, because this class of agents is very heterogeneous in many aspects; so for practical reasons, different kinds of classification have been proposed.

A first approach is to try to classify the possible biological site of action, referring to data reported in the literature (table 2) [3].

One aspect of this first classification is that, although multiple mechanisms by which mucus can be affected have been identified, the best and most predictable effects are obtained with substances that are

Table 1. Glossary of terms used in mucology [3]

Term	Definition
Bronchomucotropic	Acts directly on bronchial glands to augment their output of mucoid secretion
Bronchorrheic	Acts by nonspecific irritation or hyperosmolality to increase the transepithelial secretion of water
Ciliary excitant	Increases rate and/or effectiveness of ciliary beat
Detergent	Reduces adhesiveness of secretions to mucosal surface by surface-active effect
Diluent	Dilutes the respiratory secretions by simple addition of water
Expectorant	Acts reflexy on bronchial glands to increase their output of mucoid secretion
Fluidifier	Term used to describe drug causing increased mucous mobility through several mechanisms
Hydrating agent	Causes water to be incorporated into the structure of respiratory secretions
Liquefier	Same as mucolytic
Mucoactive	Term to indicate all drugs having a beneficial effect on respiratory secretions without specific regard to the mechanism of action
Mucolytic	Breaks up glycoproteins, other proteins, DNA and macromolecules into smaller components
Mucokinetic	Term used to describe all drugs that improve the mobilization and clearance of abnormal respiratory secretions
Mucomodifying	Same as mucoactive
Mucoregulator	Causes the synthesis of more normal biochemical components of mucus
Mucosecretolytic	Same as fluidifier
Mucospissic	Causes thickening of abnormally hypoviscous mucus
Secretolytic	Same as fluidifier
Surfactant agent	Stimulates type II alveolar cell secretion
Tensioactive	Same as detergent
Wetting agent	Same as detergent

believed to act either within the secretory cells or directly on the mucus.

A second possibility is a chemical classification, but since the chemical structures are many and varied, a chemical classification of substances that have an effect on mucus is complicated and not used very often.

Pharmacologists are more accustomed to classification by function. A first dichotomy is between drugs acting directly on mucus and those with indirect action (table 3) [3].

Table 2. Site of action of drugs acting on mucus [3]

Site of action	Mechanism involved
Central nervous system	Pituitary-adrenal axis
	Vagal inhibition or stimulation
Systemic	Hormonal control (sympathetic and parasympathetic mediators)
Within the cell	Genetic (for the synthesis of mucus glycoproteins)
	Rough endoplasmic reticulum (for synthesis of the primary polypeptide backbone)
	Golgi complex and smooth endoplasmic reticulum (glycosylation of polypeptides to form glycoproteins)
	Cell secretory apparatus (regulating the release of mucus)
	Lysosomes
Directly on mucus	Changes in physicochemical characteristics

In this case, the term 'indirect action' indicates an effect resulting in the rupture of the molecular bonds of mucoproteins. Thus, this class of drugs can be defined as agents that break the polymeric structure of mucus.

Only chemicals with free thiol groups of proteolytic enzymes can be predicted to have such an effect on mucus.

Apart from these agents, there are, at present, no defined chemical rules for synthesizing a drug with predictable therapeutic activity on mucus.

The remaining drugs have various kinds of indirect effects. Table 3 lists the different types of action of this heterogeneous group of substances on different parameters, such as mucin biochemistry adhesiveness of mucus secretions, modification of the sol layer and the gastric vagal reflex.

It is readily appreciated that some drugs, also including such traditional agents as water, hypotonic and hypertonic salt solutions, iodides, balsams and guaifenesin can have more than one mechanism of action and therefore could be placed in several classe. Pharmacological details for every drug are already known and have very recently been reviewed in a book [4], so I would like to discuss some factors that we can call 'limiting factors', which complicate our possibilities to investigate these drugs better and deeper.

Table 3. Classification of mucoactive drugs according to direct or indirect effects on bronchial secretions [3]

Direct action	Drugs breaking mucous polymers	Thiols	Cysteine[a]
			Methylcysteine[a]
			Ethylcysteine[a]
			Acetylcysteine
			α-Mercaptopropionylglycine (thiopronine)
			2-Mercaptoethanesulfonate (mesna)
		Enzymes	Trypsin, α-chymotrypsin
			Streptodornase, streptokinase
			Serratiopeptidase, sfericase, onoprose
		Other agents	Urea[a]
			Ascorbic acid[a]
			Hypertonic salt solutions[a]
			Inorganic iodides
Indirect action	Drugs modifying mucin biochemistry and mucus secretion		Bromhexine
			S-carboxymethylcysteine
			Letosteine
			Stepronine[b]
			Sobrerol
			Iodoethylene glycerol (domiodol)
			Iodopropylidene glycerol
	Drugs modifying the adhesiveness of the gel layer		Ambroxol
			Tyloxapol[a]
			Propylene glycol[a]
			Sodium ethasulfate[a]
			Sodium bicarbonate[a]
	Drugs modifying the sol layer and hydration		Water[a]
			Sodium salts[a]
			Potassuim salts[a]
	Volatile inhalants and balsams		Pinanes
			Terpenes
			Methanes
			Phenol derivatives
	Drugs stimulating gastropulmonary reflex		Ammonium chloride
			Sodium citrate
			Guaifenesin
			Ipecacuanha
	Drugs modifying bronchial gland activity		Adrenergic agents
			Cholinergic agents
			Corticosteroids
			Antihistamines
	Mucospissics		Antibiotics
			Others

Not all drugs reported are in clinical use.
[a] Topically administered.
[b] Stepronine is a prodrug for thiopronine.

From the point of view of experimental pharmacology, the main limiting factor is that we do not yet have a single experimental pharmacological model that mimicks the human pathological situation.

For instance, drugs for arthritis can be studied in experimental arthritis in the rat induced by Freund's adjuvant which almost completely mimicks a similar histological, biochemical and pathological situation in man, thus permitting a comprehensive study.

Experimentally induced bronchopneumopathies

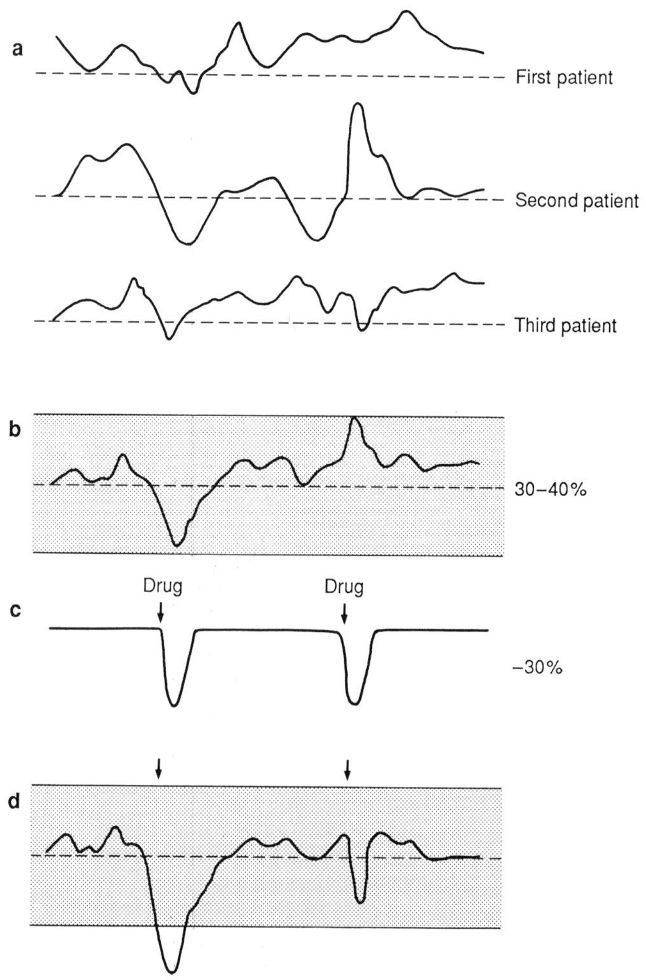

Fig. 1. a Example of random behavior of viscosity in time of expectorated mucus of different patients. **b** Window of variability (30–40%) of viscosity of expectorated mucus. **c** Reduction (–30%) of viscosity of expectorated mucus induced by a mucoactive drug. **d** Algebraic interaction of random behavior of expectorated mucus viscosity with the effect of mucoactive drug. The first arrow shows the evidence of the effect, while the second arrow shows that the noise can overlap the signal, masking the real effect.

described in different animals and produced by different techniques, are still not well standardized.

To overcome this problem which is due to the complexity and multifaced aspects of mucus secretions, experimental studies are split into different kinds of tests using different kinds of animals.

To investigate mucus production, the mouse, the rat and the rabbit are used, and the same for ciliary activity, but with addition of the chicken embryo. For mucociliary clearance, for instance, we start from the frog palate, proceeding to a fibroscopy in the sheep, and so on for the other kinds of investigations.

In each case, this means that to reach our goal of a pharmacological profile, instead of using information from one or two models, we must correlate many single data coming from heterogeneous experimental tests and conditions, and this does not facilitate uniformity of judgement.

From the point of view of clinical pharmacology, these drugs, like any other type of drugs, are used to correct pathological situation, but this gives rise to another limiting factor, a basic problem that all mucologists have to deal with and that is forgotten much too frequently: What is the definition of 'normal or physiological mucus'?

Patients clinically classified as having chronic bronchitis, according to the SEPCR-WHO classification, are the population enrolled for investigating the effectiveness of a mucoactive drug, but the pharmacologist must be aware that this clinical classification includes patients with great differences in the hypercrine and rheologic state of their mucus.

In this class, it is possible to find, for instance, patients with a sputum viscosity ≤ 5 Pa · s and patients with a sputum viscosity >60 Pa · s (which is a very dense glue).

But if we use a drug that reduces the viscosity by half, we have in the first case 2.5 or less Pa · s, which is a viscosity near to that of saliva, while in the other case we have 30 Pa · s, which is still a high viscosity. If we put together all data of this kind, we would have great difficulties in understanding the effectiveness of a mucoactive drug, because even when the patients fit the same definition of SEPCR-WHO in this single definition there are two or more subpopulations in terms of basal values of the rheological parameters. This means that a mucoactive drug can cause different responses in relation to different kinds of mucus. Therefore, the basal measures should be stratified.

Moreover, there is great interindividual and intraindividual variability in respiratory symptoms and in mucus characteristics. In chronic diseases, every patient has his own cycle of evolution, and chronic bronchopneumopathies have a cyclic course as well, with a random behavior depending on many factors, such as the different etiologic factors, the different reactive defensive responses of the respiratory airways correlated to duration of the disease, different degree of reversibility and changes in the environmental conditions.

Moreover, the classical attempts to increase the number of subjects to reduce the variability cause a new problem, because the cycles of the disease are out of phase, and have different levels of intensity from one patient to another, and, eventually, we might have a window of variability of ≥30% of the mean.

This means that if we have a drug that is able to reduce the viscosity by 30–40%, which would be a good effect, evidence of this effect can be difficult, because this kind of event can only be detected to the point at which it coincides with the curve of random fluctuation of the viscosity.

In figure 1, two different possibilities are shown; the first shows that the algebraic interaction can be evident and the second shows that the noise can overlap the signal, masking the real effect.

To try to overcome these limiting factors, double-blind studies with very narrow inclusion criteria, randomization and multicenter recruitment can be performed together with stratification in subpopulations according to the basal values of the rheologic parameters [4].

Simple randomization does not protect enough against bias or 'unfortunate allocations', so in view of the dishomogeneity of this pathology, a balanced randomization should protect better against drawbacks.

Keeping in mind these main limiting factors, which are obviously not restricted only to mucoactive drugs, but which have such a large influence on the determination of their activity, we have a possible answer to the classic question: 'Why can the same mucoactive drug be effective in one patient and ineffective in another, when both are classified as having the same lung disease?' We can also do more rational studies on the activities of this class of drugs, which are not life-saving drugs, but, at the same time, cannot be defined as simple symptomatic drugs since passive airway obstruction can by itself induce a pathology; the mucoactive drugs in this case are of 'primary' importance.

The pharmacology of mucus is not a 'receptor pharmacology', because up to now, no specific receptors governing mucus secretion have been identified, as they have been for other kinds of secretions, but further study of molecular mechanisms of mucin synthesis and excretion should provide new information about the biochemical changes induced at the molecular level by mucoactive drugs.

There is some evidence that galactosyl transferase may be a rate-limiting enzyme for the regulation of mucin glycoprotein synthesis in vivo. This finding might provide for instance a starting point for the designing of drugs for the treatment of disease states involving hypersecretion of mucus.

The antioxidant activity, the possibility to reduce bacterial adhesion to the bronchial surface or the interaction with peptides located in the lungs are other fields of research to better characterize the pharmacology of mucoactive drugs.

A last observation about the dosage and the schedule for these drugs: recently we have observed that by giving higher doses than usual for a very short period of time (only 4 days), it is possible to observe beneficial effects on rheology and mucociliary clearance that were still present 8 days after the end of treatment, i.e. twice as long as the duration of therapy.

These data are still preliminary, but indicate the persistence of a beneficial effect after the disappearance of the drug from the body, so we can postulate that there is a sort of 'post-mucoactive effect'.

If this behavior can be shown for other drugs of this class, we can use a new schedule, e.g. in chronic bronchitic patients, a 'pulse-dosing' of 4 days and then a free period of 8 days, with obvious advantages in tolerability and compliance of the patients and protection against flare-ups.

References

1 Ziment I: Historic overview of mucoactive drugs; in Braga PC, Allegra L (eds): Drugs in Bronchial Mucology. New York, Raven Press, 1989, pp 1–33.
2 Braga PC: Mucoactive drugs: Guidelines for proper experimental and clinical pharmacological studies; in Braga PC, Allegra L (eds): Drugs in Bronchial Mucology. New York, Raven Press, 1989, pp 35–58.
3 Braga PC, Ziment I, Allegra L: Classification of agents that act on bronchial mucus; in Braga PC, Allegra L (eds): Drugs in Bronchial Mucology. New York, Raven Press, 1989, pp 59–67.
4 Braga PC, Allegra L, Bossi R, Guffanti EE, Scarpazza G, Bisetti A, Spada E, Fumagalli S: Identification of subpopulations of bronchial patients for suitable therapy by a dynamic rheological test. J Clin Pharmacol 1989;9:175–182.

P.C. Braga, MD
Department of Pharmacology
Via Vanvitelli, 32
I-20129 Milano (Italy)

Respiration 1991;58(suppl 1):52–56

0025–7931/91/0587–0052 $ 2.75/0

Long-Term Oxygen Therapy for Cor Pulmonale in Patients with Chronic Obstructive Pulmonary Disease

M. Solèr, F. Michel, A.P. Perruchoud

Division of Pulmonary Diseases, Department of Internal Medicine, University Hospital, Basel, Switzerland

Key Words. Cor pulmonale · Hypertension, pulmonary arterial · Chronic obstructive lung disease · Oxygen therapy, long-term

Abstract. Besides smoking cessation, antiobstructive therapy, and the treatment of intercurrent infections, long-term oxygen therapy has had the most impressive impact on survival in patients with chronic obstructive pulmonary disease (COPD). COPD leads to a functional and anatomical obstruction of the pulmonary vascular bed, with the development of pulmonary arterial hypertension and cor pulmonale. In these patients, survival benefit from long-term oxygen therapy (LTOT) stems mainly from improved hemodynamics. However, this improvement is limited: hypoxemic COPD patients treated by LTOT have the same life expectancy as nonhypoxemic COPD patients. Practical aspects concerning the prescription and application of LTOT are discussed, with special emphasis on ambulatory oxygen and oxygen-saving techniques.

Introduction

Major determinants of prognosis in chronic obstructive pulmonary disease (COPD) are the decline in pulmonary function [1], and the development of cor pulmonale [2]. Besides smoking cessation, antiobstructive therapy, and the treatment of intercurrent infections, the introduction of long-term oxygen therapy (LTOT) has had the most impressive impact on the survival of patients with advanced COPD [3–5].

Controlled Clinical Studies: Mechanism of Action

In hypoxemic COPD patients, long-term oxygen supplementation has clearly been demonstrated to prolong survival and improve the quality of life in the large randomized controlled trials of the Nocturnal Oxygen Therapy Trial (NOTT) Group in the USA [3], and of the MRC Working Party on Long-Term Domiciliary Oxygen Therapy in the UK [4]. These studies confirmed previous findings in smaller uncontrolled trials that oxygen could improve some physiologic variables of pulmonary hemodynamics and showed that a correlation exists between the prognostic effect of oxygen treatment and the daily duration of oxygen supplementation. After the publication of these studies, Flenley summarized the findings in terms of survival effects: ‘no oxygen is bad, oxygen for some of the time is better, but oxygen for most of the time is best’. There has been nothing to add to this statement in the last few years.

These large studies (203 patients in the NOTT trial and 87 in the MRC trial) did not provide a clear answer, however, as to the mechanisms by which supplemental oxygen improves survival.

Which are the physiologic effects of oxygen supplementation for at least 12–15 h/day? In the NOTT study (nocturnal oxygen, average 12 h/day, during the hours of sleep, versus continuous oxygen, average 19 h/day), the changes directly dependent on oxygen dose were decreases in hematocrit and pulmonary vascular resistance (PVR). All patients showed a significant improvement in neuropsychological function tests and in the subjective perception of their quality of life [3]. In the MRC trial (15 h/day vs. no oxygen), in a group of patients with more advanced disease, oxygen reduced the progression of pulmonary arterial hypertension and slightly lowered the hematocrit.

Taking together all patients on LTOT, the effects of this treatment on survival and the improvement in the quality of life are impressive. LTOT had beneficial effects on PVR and hematocrit values, but there was no direct correlation between these physiologic effects of LTOT and improvement in survival. In the NOTT trial e.g., the hematocrit values decreased by 9.2% after 18 months of continuous oxygen treatment, while they were not influenced by nocturnal oxygen treatment only. The patients with the greatest benefit to survival, however, were those with low hematocrit values at the start of therapy. In addition, even if the hematocrit value was the physiologic variable critical for survival, an overall decrease of less than 10% in the hematocrit can hardly be the explanation for the improvement in survival. Similarly, after 6 months of treatment, the continuous LTOT group showed a decrease in PVR, while there was a slight increase in PVR in the group with nocturnal oxygen only, a difference which was significant. But the patients with the highest PVR at entry into the study had the highest mortality, and those with relatively low starting PVR values were those with the best survival benefit from LTOT. The detailed analysis of the hemodynamic findings in the subgroup of patients with both a hemodynamic study at entry into the trial and after 6 months of LTOT (n = 118) demonstrated a clear association of improved survival with hemodynamic response in terms of change in mean pulmonary artery pressure (PAP) over the first 6 months of treatment, after adjustment for baseline values [6]. A clear effect of LTOT on pulmonary hemodynamics was also found in a French longitudinal study in which a progressive increase in PAP was reversed during LTOT [7].

The results of these controlled studies can best be explained by the hypothesis that COPD leads to both a functional and anatomical obstruction of the pulmonary vascular bed. The consecutive development of cor pulmonale is associated with impaired survival. While hypoxic vasoconstriction, the most potent functional component, can be reversed by supplemental oxygen, occluded and destroyed vessels will not be reopened. This second component of definitely occluded vascular bed is probably best linked to pulmonary mechanics, and FEV_1 has repeatedly been shown to be the most accurate predictor of survival in COPD patients [1, 2, 8]. The specific additional effect of LTOT as compared to short periods of high FiO_2 may be a partial reversibility of structural changes such as vascular smooth muscle hypertrophy in pulmonary arterioles. It can only be speculated, therefore, that the maximal benefit from LTOT can be achieved as long as the relative contribution of functional mechanisms to the overall increase in PVR is predominant. This is also suggested by comparing the effects of LTOT between the MRC oxygen group and the nocturnal oxygen group in the NOTT trial: the patients in the MRC trial had more advanced disease, as reflected by increased pCO_2, and higher PVR and PAP values. The effects of LTOT on pulmonary hemodynamics and overall survival were similar for the two groups of patients, although the MRC patients received an average of 3 h/day more supplemental oxygen. This hypothesis is also supported by the findings of Ashutosh et al. [9] and Ashutosh and Dunsky [10] who could predict responders and nonresponders to LTOT by repeating hemodynamic measurements in patients breathing oxygen for 24 h at an FiO_2 of 28%. Patients with a decrease in the mean PAP of 5 mm Hg and more had a significantly better survival over the following 3 years than patients who showed less of a response to this short-term oxygen treatment. Patients with a good survival were also characterized by a better exercise capacity, expressed by maximal oxygen uptake. Because exercise is one of the strongest stimuli for the recruitment of additional pulmonary vascular bed, this also seems to indicate that LTOT may have its best effect on survival (and pulmonary hemodynamics) if it is initiated at a relatively early stage.

In summary, there is reason to suggest that the survival benefit from LTOT in hypoxic COPD patients mainly stems from improved pulmonary hemodynamics. However, there are still important questions unanswered. In the NOTT study, patients with continuous oxygen treatment received on average oxygen for 7 h/day longer than patients in the nocturnal oxygen group. These additional 7 h seemed to make all the difference: mortality was reduced by almost 50% in the continuous oxygen group. One might wonder, therefore, if ambulatory oxygen, during the periods of physical activity, may have more impact on survival than oxygen during the hours of rest and sleep, or whether it was simply the additional 7 h of oxygen treatment per day (50 vs. 81% of the time). This question is still not answered with certainty. Boysen et al

Table 1. Patient selection criteria for the prescription of LTOT according to the SEP Task Group [14]

A) Primary selection criteria	
Stable COPD under optimal medical therapy, no smoking	
Arterial pO_2	< 55 mm Hg (< 7.3 kPa) on at least two occasions while breathing room air (at least 1 month apart)
or	55–60 mm Hg if hematocrit above 55% or cor pulmonale present
B) Choice of investigations before considering LTOT	
Test	Indication
Clinical examination Chest X-ray Blood gases at rest Hemoglobin, hematocrit	always
Exercise testing	PaO_2 55–65 mm Hg and/or clinical suspicion of exercise-induced desaturation
Right-heart catheterization	PaO_2 > 55 mm Hg with polycythemia, sleep-related or exercise-induced desaturation
Polysomnography	PaO_2 55–65 mm Hg with polycythemia and/or cor pulmonale. Snoring in obese COPD patients

[11] and Block et al. [12] suggested that the development of cor pulmonale could be a consequence of recurrent hypoxemic periods during sleep in COPD patients with desaturation during REM sleep. Later investigations found that such desaturations were correlated with daytime CO_2 retention and were rarely found in COPD patients with normal arterial CO_2. If one hypothesizes that desaturations during sleep did not occur to an important degree in the majority of the patients in the NOTT study (who did not show daytime CO_2 retention), then one might wonder if oxygen during daytime physical exercise is the main contribution to improved survival. The analysis of the acute effects of oxygen on pulmonary hemodynamics at rest and during exercise in the NOTT patients demonstrated a greater oxygen effect on the mean PAP during exercise [6]. This question will remain unanswered because, based on the MRC trial, nocturnal oxygen treatment per se has a significant survival effect and therefore cannot be withheld from control patients in future trials. Furthermore, it is much easier to treat a patient with oxygen during the hours of sleep than during the day.

Practical Aspects

Prescription

Based on the inclusion criteria of the two large controlled clinical trials [3, 4], guidelines for the prescription and use of LTOT have been formulated and are used with little variance in many countries (table 1) [13, 14]. LTOT is still an expensive form of treatment and, in itself, causes some inconvenience. Therefore, it needs to be restricted to those patients in whom a benefit can be expected. The clear results of the NOTT and MRC trials have led to an increased acceptance and use of this therapeutic possibility in COPD patients, to the financial coverage of this treatment by health insurance companies, and to improved institutionalized oxygen supply services in many countries.

A crucial point in the selection of patients for LTOT is an optimal antiobstructive treatment prior to the beginning of oxygen therapy to make sure that the patients will not become normoxic with adequate medical treatment alone. A French study [15] demonstrated an unexpectedly great improvement during such a stabilization period of 3 months in that 30% of the patients improved their arterial oxygen tensions to a degree that they no longer fulfilled the selection criteria for LTOT.

The effectiveness of LTOT so far has been made clear for hypoxic COPD patients fulfilling the abovementioned inclusion criteria. However, there is little evidence to support a similar effect of LTOT on other forms of chronic lung disease, such as fibrosis. In these patients, oxygen therapy has to be prescribed based on its symptomatic effect.

Technical Aspects

Domiciliary nocturnal oxygen therapy can easily be performed with a stationary oxygen source, nasal prongs, and long oxygen supply tubing. This relatively inexpensive and noninvasive form of LTOT is accepted by most patients.

Theoretically, three types of oxygen sources are available: liquid oxygen in stationary canisters, electrically powered oxygen concentrators, and compressed oxygen gas in tanks. In most cases the oxygen concentrator is the cheapest and most convenient type of stationary oxygen source, requiring only electrical power supply. It has a limited concentrating capacity for oxygen, however, and at flow rates of 4 l/min reaches oxygen concentrations of just around 85% and lower [16, 17].

The important step in terms of survival for the continuous oxygen treatment group in the NOTT study was the ambulatory used of oxygen accounting for some of the extra hours on oxygen. This step, however, is technically more difficult, and has a greater influence on the patients daily life.

One problem with ambulatory oxygen is the oxygen capacity of the portable container determining the range of mobility away from the stationary source. It is limited by the weight of the container, which should not restrict physical activities. Liquid oxygen containers have the best weight/oxygen capacity ratio, but liquid oxygen is more expensive than the other forms of oxygen supply. In this context, oxygen-saving devices come into play, which have been demonstrated to reduce oxygen needs (and the cost of treatment) without negative influence on arterial pO_2 levels. Basically, they can consist of reservoir systems designed to collect the continuously flowing oxygen during expiration and apnea, and to deliver transiently larger oxygen volumes at the beginning of inspiration, or of demand systems, interrupters to control oxygen flow from the source, opening only during inspiration [18].

In the ambulatory use of supplemental oxygen, cosmetic aspects of oxygen application become more important. A clear cosmetical improvement was achieved with the introduction of transtracheal oxygen catheters [19, 20]. However, this advantage has to be weighed against the potential complications of this invasive approach. Mucus balls forming at the distal end of the cannula, local infections, displacement, and hemoptysis have been reported [19, 20]. Their incidence, however, seems to be low if the transtracheal catheter is carefully cleaned and regularly changed. In the studies published so far, the acceptance of this device was excellent [19, 20]. Patients with transtracheal catheters not only demonstrated the expected effects of continuous oxygen treatment but also less days of hospitalization, which was probably a consequence of the closer medical follow-up. Transtracheal catheters also help resolve the problem of oxygen saving because the reservoir function of the trachea and upper airways, filled by continuously flowing oxygen during endexspiration and apnea, leads to a bolus of oxygen in the first portion of inspired air allowing to reduce the oxygen flow from the portable source by approximately 50%. The most significant oxygen savings can be achieved by combining transtracheal delivery with a demand valve system. With these measures, even compressed gas cylinders can be used to allow a reasonable duration of ambulatory activity.

Conclusion

LTOT has become a widely used and highly effective treatment in patients with advanced COPD and hypoxemia. Its effect on survival is impressive, but one should not forget the other, and probably more important, determinant, i.e. the degree of airway obstruction. At its best, LTOT seems to improve the prognosis of hypoxemic COPD patients such that they have the same life expectancy as nonhypoxic COPD patients of the same age with the same degree of airway obstruction [1].

References

1 Anthonisen NR, Wright EC, Hodgkin JE, IPPB trial group: Prognosis in chronic obstructive pulmonary disease. Am Rev Respir Dis 1986;133:14–20.

2 Traver GA, Cline MG, Burrows B: Predictors of mortality in chronic obstructive pulmonary disease: A 15-year follow-up study. Am Rev Respir Dis 1979;119:895–902.
3 NOTT Group: Continuous or nocturnal oxygen therapy in hypoxemic chronic obstructive lung disease. Ann Intern Med 1980;93:391–398.
4 MRC Working Party: Long-term domiciliary oxygen therapy in chronic hypoxic cor pulmonale complicating chronic bronchitis and emphysema. Lancet 1981;i:681–686.
5 Anthonisen NR: Long-term oxygen therapy. Ann Intern Med 1983;99:519–527.
6 Timms RM, Khaja FU, Williams GW, NOTT Group: Hemodynamic response to oxygen therapy in chronic obstructive pulmonary disease. Ann Intern Med 1985;102:29-36.
7 Weitzenblum E, Sautegeau A, Ehrhart M, Mammosser M, Pelletier A: Long-term oxygen therapy can reverse the progression of pulmonary hypertension in patients with chronic obstructive pulmonary disease. Am Rev Respir Dis 1985;131: 493–498.
8 Cooper CB, Waterhouse J, Howard P: Twelve-year clinical study of patients with hypoxic cor pulmonale given long-term domiciliary oxygen therapy. Thorax 1987;42:105–110.
9 Ashutosh K, Mead G, Dunsky M: Early effects of oxygen administration and prognosis in chronic obstructive pulmonary disease and cor pulmonale. Am Rev Respir Dis 1983;127: 399–404.
10 Ashutosh K, Dunsky M: Noninvasive tests for responsiveness of pulmonary hypertension to oxygen. Chest 1987;92:393–399.
11 Boysen AG, Block AJ, Wynne JW, Hunt LA, Flick MR: Nocturnal pulmonary hypertension in patients with chronic obstructive pulmonary disease. Chest 1979;76:536–542.
12 Block AJ, Boysen PG, Wynne JW: The origins of cor pulmonale: A hypothesis. Chest 1979;75:109–110.
13 Petty TL, Snider GL: Second Oxygen Consensus Conference Report: Further recommendations for prescribing and supplying long-term oxygen therapy. Am Rev Respir Dis 1988;138: 745–747.
14 SEP Task Group: Recommendations for long-term oxygen therapy. Eur Respir J 1989;2:160–164.
15 Levi-Valensi P, Weitzenblum E, Pedinelli JL, Racineux JL, Duwoos H: Three-month follow-up of arterial blood gas determinations in candidates for long-term oxygen therapy. Am Rev Respir Dis 1986;133:547–551.
16 Johns DP, Rochford PD, Streeton JA: Evaluation of six oxygen concentrators. Thorax 1985;40:806–810.
17 Gould GA, Scott W, Mayhurst MD, Flenley DC: Technical and clinical assessment of oxygen concentrators. Thorax 1985;40: 811–816.
18 Tiep BL, Lewis MI: Oxygen conservation and oxygen conserving devices in chronic lung disease. A review. Chest 1987;92: 263–272.
19 Heimlich HJ, Carr GC: The micro-trach. A seven-year experience with transtracheal oxygen therapy. Chest 1989;95: 1008–1012.
20 Christopher KL, Spofford BT, Petrun MD, McCarthy DC, Goodman JR, Petty TL: A program for transtracheal oxygen delivery: Assessment of safety and efficacy. Ann Intern Med 1987;107:802–808.

Prof. A.P. Perruchoud
Division of Pulmonary Diseases
Department of Internal Medicine
University Hospital
CH-4031 Basel (Switzerland)

Author Index

Subject Index

Contributions to Oncology/Beiträge zur Onkologie
(ISSN 0250–3220), **Vol. 35**
Series Editors: J.H. Holzner, Wien; W. Queisser, Mannheim

Ifosfamide in the Treatment of Lung Cancer

Editor: D.K. Hossfeld

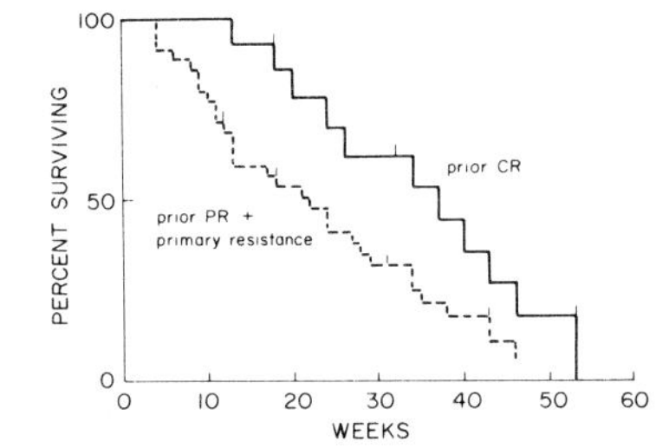

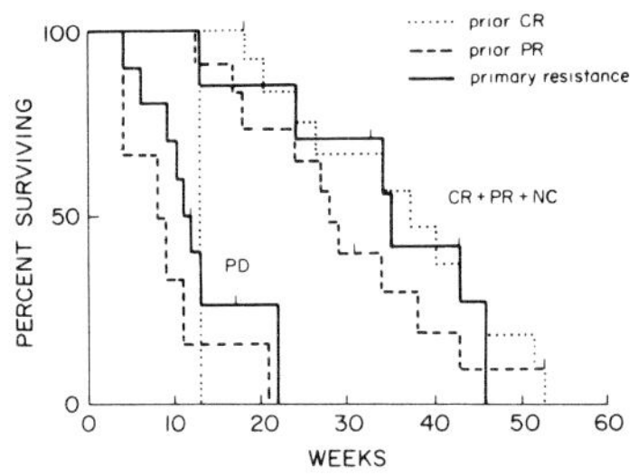

A thorough and expert evaluation

While ifosfamide is one of the most active drugs in the treatment of lung cancer, results in both small cell and non-small cell lung cancer are still far from being satisfactory. This is the first book to provide a comprehensive overview of the applications and results of ifosfamide therapy in patients with both cancer types. The contributions, selected from the 19th German Cancer Congress, report the results of clinical trials and discuss the latest efforts to improve the effectiveness of chemotherapy in lung cancer.
Allowing a comparison of the experiences of an impressive number of international groups, this is a unique single source of information on this widely-used drug ideal for clinical oncologists, internists and pulmonary specialists.

Contents

Fields of Interest
Oncology; Pneumology, Respiratory System; Pharmacology, Pharmaceutics; Chemotherapy

Contributions to Oncology/Beiträge zur Onkologie, Vol. 35
Ifosfamide in the Treatment of Lung Cancer
Satellite Symposium of the 19th German Cancer Congress, Frankfurt a.M., February 1988
Editor: Hossfeld, D.K. (Hamburg)
VIII + 154 p., 29 fig., 46 tab., hard cover, 1989
SFr. 75.– / DM 90.– / £ 32.60 / US$ 60.00
US$ price for USA, £ price for UK only (subject to change)
ISBN 3–8055–5199–1